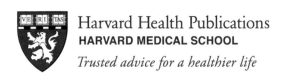

Harvard Health Publications
HARVARD MEDICAL SCHOOL
Trusted advice for a healthier life

Dear Reader,

Good for you for picking up this Special Health Report. That means you realize the importance of strength and power training—and you're doing something about it. Most people are familiar with the recommendation to get 150 minutes of moderate aerobic activity a week. But they often overlook the recommendation to do muscle-strengthening exercises two or three times a week, too. According to the latest data from the National Center for Health Statistics, only 25% of American adults do strength training twice a week.

Strength training offers benefits beyond buff biceps or six-pack abs—payoffs that you just can't get with aerobic exercise, despite its many virtues. It is the type of exercise that will do the most to keep your muscles and bones strong as you age. Strong, powerful muscles will keep you fit, so you can enjoy your favorite activities like hiking, skiing, or gardening for longer. They'll make keeping up with your kids (or grandkids) easier. They may even help your golf or tennis game and make it easier to lose weight or stay slim. And if you have certain health concerns, strength training may help with those issues, too. Studies show that strength training can help prevent or control conditions as varied as arthritis and type 2 diabetes.

While strength training is a familiar concept to most people, power training, which builds both strength and speed, may be new to you. There is overlap between the two, but think of it this way: strength training may help you lift your suitcase into the overhead bin, but power training can help you react quickly to catch a bag that falls from the bin.

This report offers four strength and power routines that give you total-body, multi-muscle moves and also improve your balance. You'll begin with workouts using dumbbells and your own body weight or resistance bands. Then you can add medicine balls or kettlebells to take it to the next level. Finally, there's a section on plyometrics, or jumping exercises, that you can incorporate into any of the workouts to rev up your calorie burn and maximize muscle power. In every workout, we offer easier and harder options, so you can adjust the workouts to your own strength and fitness level. (Note: While this program is highly adaptable, we recommend that you start with our earlier report, *Strength and Power Training for Older Adults*, if you are over 65 or have health problems such as heart disease, diabetes, or joint or bone problems.)

Whatever your age, the strength and power training routines in this report will help you look and feel younger and more vital. Above all, we hope you will have fun working out. We do!

Sincerely,

Elizabeth Pegg Frates, M.D.
Medical Editor

Michele Stanten
Fitness Consultant

The basics: Strength training, power training, and your muscles

The last time you visited the doctor, you may have received a list of recommendations to improve your health—consume less salt, lose 10 pounds, exercise regularly. But chances are, your doctor didn't mention strength training or power training. Most people don't give their muscles enough thought, except maybe when they pull one. But just like your heart and brain, muscles play a vital role in your life. And how you treat them now can make a big difference in how much fun you will have for years to come.

Sure, strong muscles can help you unscrew a stuck lid, but they also power your tennis or golf swing, put spring in your step to dance the night away, and keep you going whether you're hiking up a mountain or crossing the finish line. Stronger muscles also make more mundane tasks like carrying groceries and hoisting suitcases easier. But if you neglect your muscles, you will find that these activities require more effort as you age.

In your mid-30s, you start to lose muscle mass at a rate of 1% to 2% a year, and strength decreases by 1.5% a year. That may not sound like much, but these little changes add up in your 40s and 50s and may contribute to achy joints, an increased risk of injury, and an expanding waistline. The less muscle mass you have, the fewer calories you burn throughout the day, which primes your body to gain weight.

As you reach your 60s and 70s, muscle loss accelerates to 3% a year. This makes everyday activities harder, so you are likely to become less active. Eventually, even simple tasks such as climbing stairs, walking, and just getting out of a chair become more difficult.

However, these changes are not an inevitable part of aging. Strength and power training are some of the best tools you have to keep looking and feeling young. They may even help keep your brain fit. A 2016 study of British twins (ages 43 to 73) in the journal *Geron-*

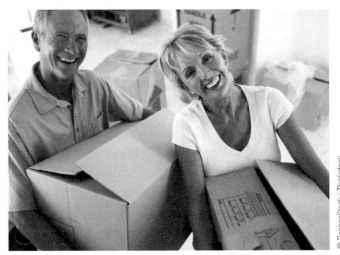

Building stronger muscles isn't just about showing off at the gym. Stronger muscles make mundane tasks like carrying groceries and hoisting heavy boxes easier. If you neglect your muscles, you will find that these activities become more difficult as you age.

tology found that, among 324 twin pairs, those with the most muscle strength maintained the best performance on memory and cognitive tests over a 10-year period—and had greater brain volume on brain scans.

Before delving into all the benefits of muscle-strengthening exercise, it helps to review what strength training is, how power training is different, and how these exercises affect your muscles. You'll also learn how muscles work and how aging and inactivity contribute to the loss of muscle strength and power over the years.

Strength training: The traditional approach

The classic image of strength training is body builders with bulging muscles lifting weights. But strength training is much broader than that. Strength training is any exercise that builds muscle by harnessing resistance—that is, an opposing force that muscles must strain against. It is also known as resistance training, progressive resistance training, weight training, or weight lifting. There are many ways to supply resistance. You can use your own body weight, free weights such as dumbbells, elasticized bands, or specialized machines. Other options include medicine balls, kettlebells, and weighted ropes.

No matter what kind of resistance you use, strength training builds muscle. This not only makes you stronger, but also increases your muscles' endurance, making activities like running a marathon or even standing for hours along a parade route easier. And it doesn't take as much work as you might think to start seeing results. In a study of about 1,600 men and women who lifted weights two or three times a week, participants gained an average of three pounds of lean weight (muscle) in 10 weeks. When you consider that you've probably been losing muscle since about your mid-30s, you can see how important it is to build and maintain muscle mass as you age.

The benefits are not limited to your muscles. These exercises can strengthen your bones as well. When your muscles contract, they pull on the bones to which they're attached, and this force stimulates your body to reinforce the bones with added minerals. Note that the only bones that benefit are those attached to the working muscles, which is one reason why it's important to do a full-body workout that exercises all the major muscle groups. The workouts in this report will do that.

Power training: A complementary approach

Another type of training, known as power training, is proving to be just as important as traditional strength training in helping to maintain or rebuild muscles and strength—maybe even more important.

As the name suggests, power training is aimed at increasing power, which is the product of both strength and speed, reflecting how quickly you can exert force to produce the desired movement. Thus, faced with a mountain hike, you may have enough strength to reach the summit. But can you keep up with the younger members of your hiking group? Power, not just strength and cardio fitness, can get you

up the steep inclines quickly and safely. By helping you react swiftly if you trip over a root or lose your balance on loose rocks, power can actually prevent falls.

To develop power, you need to add speed as you work against resistance. You can do this by performing traditional strength exercises such as push-ups or biceps curls at a faster pace, while maintaining good form. Plyometrics, such as jumping exercises, also build muscle power. The rapid acceleration as you leap into the air and then the rapid deceleration as you land increase your ability to produce explosive power—for example, darting across the street when a car ignores the crosswalk sign or chasing after a toddler headed for trouble. Exercises such as medicine ball throws increase upper-body power, so you're better able to catch a box of oatmeal if it falls from a shelf.

Power training may be even more important than strength training because muscle power declines at more than twice the rate that strength does as you age—as much as 3.5% a year for power compared with 1.5% for strength. That's why some doctors, physical therapists, and personal trainers are now combining the swift moves of power training with slower, more deliberate strength training exercises, as do the workouts in this report, to reap the benefits of both activities.

A look at muscles and movement

Any voluntary movement in the body is made possible by skeletal muscles, which are attached to bone. The body boasts more than 600 skeletal muscles that enable you to walk, twist, swing your arms, turn your head, flex your feet, wiggle your toes, and more. Figure 1 shows the muscles you'll be exercising with the workouts in this report.

Some of these muscles—like the biceps and triceps in your upper arms—are muscles you've heard about your whole life. But a well-rounded strength program works major and minor muscle groups throughout your body. This is especially important if your current exercise routine is limited to some of the most popular cardio workouts like walking, running, or cycling. These activities focus on the lower body, so muscles in your upper body are often neglected. Strength training balances things out by providing a workout

Figure 1: The muscles you'll be working

For each exercise in this report, you will see a line indicating "Muscles worked." The diagram below shows where most of those muscles are located. However, there are some exceptions. Certain muscles we name in the exercises are not visible here, since they are underneath other muscles. The rhomboids are located underneath the trapezius muscles in the back and link the shoulder blades to the spinal column. The erector spinae muscles are up and down the spine. The internal obliques lie underneath the external obliques. And the psoas major and transverse abdominis lie deep beneath the lower portion of the rectus abdominis.

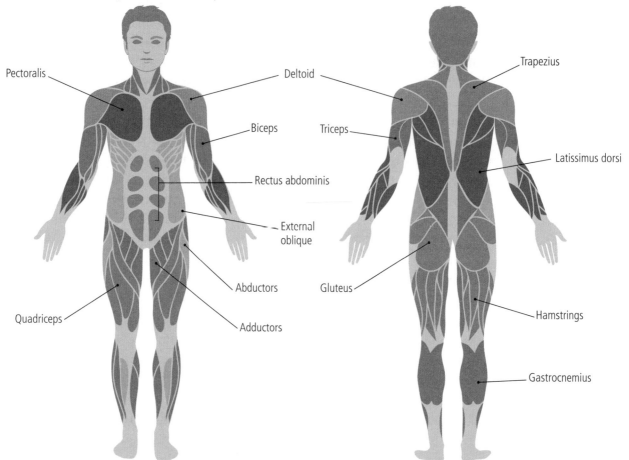

© kowalska-art | Thinkstock

for the total body, including the core muscles in your abdomen and back. The core is the sturdy central link connecting your upper and lower body and, as such, assists everything from swinging a golf club to bending to pick up a package. When muscles throughout the body remain strong and balanced, you can perform at a high level with less risk of injury.

When you're young, it's easy to perform tasks or play sports despite muscle imbalances, but this changes as you age—and it's never ideal, no matter how old you are. Any time you move, your muscles are applying force. To balance this force properly, different sets of muscles move in opposition to one another. So, as you walk up stairs, the quadriceps muscles on the front of your thighs act as agonists, meaning that they initiate the movement. On the back of your thighs, the hamstring muscles work as antagonists, meaning that they help to control the movement. This synergistic relationship is the reason you need to exercise both sets of muscles; otherwise, you will create an imbalance in strength that can increase your chances of being injured, especially as you get older.

For a well-functioning, injury-free body, it's also important to work some of the deeper and smaller muscles. For example, the abductor and adductor muscles in your legs and hips are vital to keeping you upright as you walk or run, so you want to keep them performing at a high level. The routines in this report involve these and other small, deep muscles along with the more superficial ones that provide nice definition. Table 1 explains the functions of the different muscles that are targeted in the workouts.

Muscles in motion

As you perform the exercises in this report, your muscles will engage in three types of action. Paying attention to what your muscles are doing as you execute a move will improve your form and technique, so there's less chance of injury.

Concentric action occurs when muscles exert force and move joints while shortening. When people think of using their muscles, this is usually what comes to mind—for example, flexing an arm to show off the biceps muscle in the upper arm. This is the same type of motion you would use when bending your arms to lift a bag of groceries out of the back of the car or hoisting the bag up to the kitchen counter.

Eccentric action occurs when muscles exert force and move joints while *lengthening*. As you slowly lower your grocery bag, the biceps muscles lengthen while producing force, so that you lower the object in a controlled manner rather than simply letting it drop. According to the American Academy of Sports Medicine, eccentric strength is especially important for maintaining balance, mobility, and everyday functions.

Isometric (static) action creates force, too, but muscles don't shorten or lengthen much and joints do not move. If you push against a wall, for example,

Table 1: Know your muscles

A well-rounded strength training program works all the major muscle groups. These are the major muscle groups in your body and the actions and tasks they perform. The workouts in this Special Health Report will ensure that you train all of these key muscles.

BODY PART	MUSCLE	ACTION	EXAMPLE
Shoulders and arms	Deltoid	Moves your entire arm at the shoulder joint	Waving arm overhead
	Biceps	Bends your arm at the elbow joint	Raising a glass to drink
	Triceps	Extends your arm at the elbow joint	Pushing up a window
Back	Trapezius	Moves your shoulder and shoulder blade	Shrugging
	Rhomboid	Moves your shoulder blade	Starting a lawnmower
	Latissimus dorsi	Pulls your arm down	Pulling down a window
	Erector spinae	Extends your spine	Standing tall
Front of torso	Pectoralis	Moves your arm up, down, in, and out	Pushing something away from you, lifting a child off the floor
	Rectus abdominis	Bends your torso	Sitting up in bed
	Transverse abdominis	Stabilizes lower spine and pelvis	Pulling your belly in
	Internal and external obliques	Rotate your torso	Dancing the twist
	Psoas major	Bends and rotates your leg	Marching
Hips, buttocks, and legs	Gluteus	Extends your leg behind you	Standing up from a chair
	Quadriceps	Extends your lower leg at the knee joints	Kicking a ball
	Hamstrings	Pull your heel toward your buttock	Running
	Abductors	Move your leg away from the midline of your body	Swinging your leg out to the side
	Adductors	Move your leg toward or across the midline of your body	Kicking your leg across your body
	Gastrocnemius	Point your toes	Rising up onto your toes

or try to lift an object that is far too heavy for you, you'll feel your arm muscles tense. But since your muscles can't generate enough force to lift the object or shift the wall, they stay in their usual position instead of shortening.

Here's what all of that means in practical terms. Concentric and eccentric muscle actions create movement, whether you are lifting weights, jogging, or simply walking across a room. As you perform an exercise, the muscle targeted by that exercise will alternate between concentric and eccentric actions. For example, as you lift and lower a weight, your biceps will first shorten (concentric action), then lengthen (eccentric action). The opposing muscles, the triceps, also do both, but in the reverse order—lengthening as the biceps contracts and vice versa. Because your muscles work in tandem, as explained earlier, both muscle groups get some benefit, but the primary movers—in this case, your biceps—get the most strengthening.

Though most people tend to think of the concentric phase of the exercise as the whole point of that exercise, both phases are important. Slowing down the eccentric phase of an exercise has been shown to improve strength gains. However, you are also more likely to experience soreness a day or so after training in this manner. The strength workouts in this report use a tempo that achieves maximum strength gains with minimal soreness.

As for isometric exercise, your core muscles perform this type of contraction when you are doing exercises like a lunge or a standing overhead press in order to stabilize you so you don't fall over. Isometric muscle actions result in very little movement, such as when a soldier stands at attention, but they are essential for maintaining your balance.

Muscle physiology

A muscle seems like a simple thing. But a single muscle may have from 10,000 to over a million muscle fibers (also known as muscle cells). Inside muscle fibers, you will find protein, glycogen (sugar), and fat stores that provide energy for muscle contraction. In order for the fibers to function together as a unit, they are grouped together in small bundles known as fasciculi (see Figure 2).

Still, a muscle could not contract without nerve impulses. A single nerve cell, or motor neuron, directs activity in a specific group of muscle fibers. Together, this grouping of nerve cell and muscle fibers is called a motor unit. If a given nerve cell commands few muscle fibers, the motor unit marshals less force; the more fibers a nerve cell controls, the greater the force the unit exerts.

When nerve impulses originating in the brain shoot along neural pathways toward a muscle, they trigger a complex set of chemical reactions that cause contractile proteins (myofilaments) deep in the muscle to slide over each other, generating force. Movement occurs when that force ripples through the muscle structure to the tendons, which in turn tug on the bones. Essentially, the bunching muscles act like strings that make a puppet spring to life.

Figure 2: An in-depth look at muscle

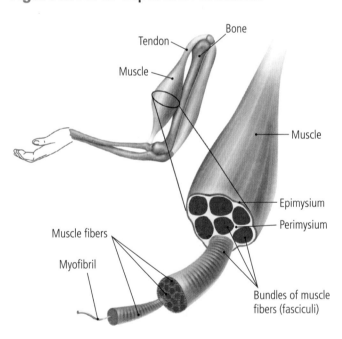

Your muscles are joined to bone by cords of tissue known as tendons and are covered in connective tissue known as the epimysium. If you could look inside your muscles, you would find that they are composed of small bundles of muscle fibers, known as fasciculi. These bundles are surrounded by connective tissue, known as the perimysium. One muscle may have anywhere from 10,000 to more than a million muscle fibers. In turn, each muscle fiber consists of hundreds to thousands of tiny, interlocking strands called myofibrils.

Strength and power training exercises push muscle beyond its usual capacity. Muscles grow in response to this stimulus because the exercises increase the production of new muscle protein. When this cycle occurs repeatedly, muscles become stronger, muscle mass increases, and muscles may become visibly larger, particularly in men. Women can develop more shapely arms and legs, but they are unlikely to develop big, bulky muscles unless they spend hours a day in the gym, because their bodies have far less of the male hormone testosterone, which contributes to muscle bulk. Interestingly, even if there is no muscle growth, strength and power training enhance the ability of the nervous system to activate motor units.

Slow-twitch and fast-twitch fibers

Most skeletal muscles have two main types of muscle fibers: slow-twitch and fast-twitch. Usually, a combination of these types gets called into service when you exercise. Slow-twitch fibers function best during low-intensity activities, when they can be supplied with oxygen. These fibers can keep working for long periods of time and are called upon first for most activities, including aerobic activities such as walking, swimming, biking, or jogging. During anaerobic activity (rapid, high-intensity exercise in which your body is unable to meet the muscles' significantly higher oxygen demands—for example, short bouts of sprinting, jumping, or scrambling up a hill), fast-twitch fibers step into the breach to create bursts of power. Generally speaking, classic strength training is better for developing slow-twitch fibers, while power training favors the fast-twitch fibers. But in fact, you usually use both to varying degrees when you exercise.

Studies show that functional activities—that is, activities that people do in their daily lives—also call on both kinds of fibers. Take something as mundane as washing the dishes. The slow-twitch fibers act during most of the slow-paced activity of scrubbing, rinsing, and drying. But when you reach overhead to put away a heavy dish, the fast-twitch fibers are recruited because you are doing something that needs a short but more intense burst of power. ▼

What strength and power training can do for you

No matter how old—or how young—you are, strength and power training can offer benefits. Studies in children and young people, some as little as 8 years old, have found improvements in sports performance (among athletes), body composition (among those who are overweight or obese), and physical and psychological well-being (across all categories). And benefits continue across your life span, even into your 80s and 90s. Some research has included subjects as old as 97 and has shown that strength training helps the elderly stay independent longer.

One of the reasons that strength and power training are so potent, especially as you get older, is their ability to curb muscle loss and build new muscle. As mentioned earlier, muscle loss begins around age 35. On average, adults who don't do regular strength training can expect to lose 4 to 6 pounds of muscle per decade.

If you're trying to lose weight, that might sound appealing, but it's not a good thing. First, most people don't see the number on the scale go down because of muscle loss, since they are usually simultaneously replacing that firm, compact muscle with bigger, lumpy fat. That's why you may notice your pants feeling snug even if the scale hasn't changed. Second, muscles fuel metabolism, so the less muscle a body has, the slower its metabolism, meaning it's burning fewer calories throughout the day—exactly the opposite of what you want it to do. And if you're trying to lose weight by cutting calories, you're likely losing even more muscle.

But strength training can counteract this effect. According to a research review in *The Journal of Sports Medicine and Physical Fitness*, on average, 27% of the weight lost by dieting is muscle. Combining dieting with cardio exercise cut muscle loss in half. But when participants combined dieting and resistance training, *all* of the pounds lost were fat.

The more muscle you have and the stronger your muscles are, the more benefits you'll get, even beyond weight loss. You'll develop a slimmer, firmer figure. You'll be more active. You'll get more out of your cardio exercise because you'll be able to go faster and last longer. Strength training can even improve your golf game. After 10 weeks of training, 29 amateur female golfers (average age 58) improved their drive speed and distance, according to a study in the journal *Physical Therapy in Sport*.

Moreover, there are specific health benefits to strength and power training, such as better blood sugar control and a slowing of bone loss.

Given that you only need to put in an hour or so of effort every week, that's a lot of benefits. This chapter delves into more of the research on strength and power training, starting with power training, which is newer to the scene and has been studied less extensively.

Health benefits of power training

Football players, high jumpers, and other athletes have long used power training, particularly with weighted vests, to help improve performance. Many studies have documented not only improvements in performance with power training, but also reductions in injuries.

For non-athletes, there aren't as many studies on power training, but research in this area is growing, especially among older adults, and it has already yielded promising results. The documented benefits include preventing falls, preserving and enhancing physical functioning, and improving quality of life.

There may also be benefits for people with certain health problems. One small study tested three types of exercise—strength training, power training, and stretching—on people with osteoarthritis of the knee. After 12 weeks of exercise, participants in all three groups had better function and less pain, but those in the power training group registered the greatest gains in strength, power, and walking speed. A second small study found no gains in speed, but did confirm reductions in pain and improvements in tasks of daily living.

Power training can even help if you have severe joint pain requiring a joint replacement—something that more people are opting for today at younger ages. In one Danish study, 40 patients did power training twice a week for 10 weeks before undergoing hip replacement surgery. Following their conditioning, the power trainers reported less pain and stiffness and improved daily functioning, along with gains in muscle power, compared with another group of 40 patients who did no exercise. The conditioning did not cause the participants to delay or cancel their joint replacements, but the researchers speculate that this level of improvement might cause people with less severe osteoarthritis to delay surgery. The improvements noted with power training might also help the power trainers fare better after surgery—something the researchers are examining in another part of the study that is not yet complete.

Plyometrics, such as jumping exercises or explosive push-ups, are a type of power training that can benefit both sports performance and general health. They can improve your tennis game by increasing your reaction time and giving you more powerful push-off as you go after the ball. These high-impact exercises can also benefit your bones. Over 16 weeks, women ages 25 to 50 increased bone density in their hips by doing 10 to 20 jumps twice a day, according to a study published in the *American Journal of Health Promotion*.

Health benefits of strength training

Scientists have long known that strength training has a positive impact on your body. Conditions as varied as back pain, heart disease, arthritis, osteoporosis, diabetes, obesity, and insomnia can be partly managed by strength training and other exercise regimens.

But what is the relative importance of strength training versus aerobic workouts? Relatively few large, long-term studies have examined this question. Some things are clear, however.

Strong muscles never sleep. While strength training doesn't burn as many calories as the same amount of time jogging or swimming, it does appear to have a bigger afterburn. Technically called "excess post-exercise oxygen consumption," this refers to the extra calories you burn after an exercise session as your body returns to its normal state. Generally, the higher the intensity and the longer the workout, the longer this excess calorie burn lasts. That means the more strength training you do, the more calories you can burn even after you put the weights down. One study found that on non-exercise days following strength training, participants burned on average an extra 240 calories a day through everyday activities—a significantly higher amount than on days following cardio.

Other studies confirm that strength training can increase your metabolic rate (the rate at which your body converts energy stores to working energy) by up to 15%. This means you burn more calories, even while you're sitting or sleeping.

Strength training can also boost your self-esteem. Seeing changes in your body, often more quickly than with cardio exercise, can increase your self-confidence as well. Studies in both men and women document the psychological benefits. For example, in a Montana State University study, 341 women ages 23 to 87 did a strength training class twice a week for about 10 weeks. As a result, they significantly improved their body image, became more active throughout the day, and reported enjoying physical activity more.

Here are some other ways in which strength training improves specific health conditions.

Slowing bone loss

As with loss of muscle mass, bone strength starts to decline earlier than you might imagine, slipping at an average rate of 1% per year after age 40. About 10.2 million Americans have osteoporosis, which is defined by weak and porous bones, and another 43 million are at risk for it.

Numerous studies have shown that weight-bearing exercise can play a role in slowing bone loss, and several show it can even build bone. Activities that put stress on bones stimulate extra deposits of calcium and nudge bone-forming cells into action. The tugging and pushing on bone that occur during strength and power training provide the stress. The result is stronger, denser bones.

Even weight-bearing aerobic exercise, like walking or running, can help your bones, but there are a couple of caveats. Generally, higher-impact activities have a more pronounced effect on bone than lower-impact aerobics. Velocity is also a factor; jogging or fast-paced aerobics will do more to strengthen bone than more leisurely movement. And keep in mind that only those bones that bear the load of the exercise will benefit. For example, walking or running protects only the bones in your lower body, including your hips.

By contrast, a well-rounded strength training program that works out all the major muscle groups can benefit practically all of your bones. Of particular interest, it targets bones of the hips, spine, and wrists, which, along with the ribs, are the sites most likely to fracture. Also, by enhancing strength and stability, resistance workouts reduce the likelihood of falls, which can lead to fractures.

Improving insulin sensitivity

About 29 million people in the United States have diabetes, and 86 million people have prediabetes. If you have diabetes, strength training can help you better control your blood sugar levels—and if you don't have the condition, strength training can reduce your risk of developing type 2 diabetes (the most common form of the disease) by making the body more sensitive to insulin and improving blood sugar control. Skeletal muscle serves as a reservoir for glucose, penning up sugar not immediately needed for fuel in the form of glycogen and doling it out as necessary. The more muscle you have, the more efficiently your body can sop up circulating blood sugar.

While aerobic exercise provides more protection against diabetes than strength training does, the best protection comes when you do both types of exercise. According to a Harvard University analysis of more than 32,000 men in the Health Professionals Follow-up Study, men who did 150 minutes of cardio a week reduced their risk of developing type 2 diabetes by 52%. Those who did an equal amount of strength training cut their risk by 34%. But doing both cardio and strength training for a total of 150 minutes a week—so no extra time needed—reduced their risk by 59%. Similar research in women showed a 40% reduction.

And you get benefits after just one workout. Research shows that a single cardio or strength session speeds the rate at which glucose enters the muscles. Note that the effect dissipates in two to four days, however, unless the activity is repeated. Regular workouts also help the body remain sensitive to insulin rather than succumbing to the creeping insulin resistance that often develops as people get older.

When diabetes does develop, strength training can help control it. One study of older adults with type 2 diabetes found that four months of strength training improved blood sugar control so much that seven out of 10 volunteers were able to reduce their dosage of diabetes medicine. The evidence supporting strength training's effect on diabetes is so compelling that the American Diabetes Association recommends that anyone with diabetes should do at least two strength workouts a week.

Even when insulin is not being produced in normal amounts by the body—as is the case with type 1 diabetes—lowering blood sugar through strength training can reduce the amount of injected insulin a person needs to keep blood sugar under control.

Easing joint pain

Strong muscles support and protect your joints, easing pain and stiffness and reducing your risk of developing osteoarthritis. In this form of arthritis, which can show up in your 40s or 50s, the cartilage that cushions your joints gradually wears away. But when strong muscles contract, they take pressure off the joints, reducing this kind of wear and tear. For instance, a study published in the journal *Arthritis and Rheumatology* suggested that greater quadriceps strength reduces cartilage loss in the knee. Without strong quadriceps, the joint bears the brunt of the impact from walking, running, or other weight-bearing activities.

Strength training may also enhance range of motion in many joints, so you'll be able to bend and reach with greater ease. In a randomized controlled study of 32 older men, after 16 weeks of workouts, men doing strength training alone or combined with cardiovascular training had significantly greater range of motion in all five of the joints tested than men who remained inactive. Among those doing just cardiovascular activities, range of motion improved in only one of the joints that were tested.

If you do develop osteoarthritis, strength training can ease pain and improve quality of life. In one study, published in 2015, older women who had either knee osteoarthritis or a knee replacement did strength training twice a week for 13 weeks. By the end of the study, the women had improved their ability to walk, climb stairs, and balance. A study in *Arthritis Care Research* also found that people with knee osteoarthritis who did power training reduced pain and improved their ability to function.

People with rheumatoid arthritis can also benefit, since muscle weakness is common among those with this illness. One study reported that moderate or high-intensity strength training was more effective at increasing or maintaining muscle strength than low-intensity programs. A key to reaping long-term benefits, though, was consistency with the training program.

Other conditions

There are many more conditions that may benefit from regular strength training. Here are a few. (Research on power training for these problems is still in its infancy.)

Depression. Strength training may help with mild to moderate depression by restoring lost abilities, which can boost confidence and open up new options for pleasurable activities; it may also alleviate dependence on others. One study of 60 older adults with depression found that high-intensity strength training was more effective at reducing depressive symptoms than low-intensity strength training, so choose challenging weights and keep working out regularly. Combining exercise with therapy or with both therapy and medication may yield the best results.

Cancer. Despite improvements, most cancer treatments still have unpleasant side effects such as fatigue, physical discomfort, impaired sleep, and emotional distress, which can impair quality of life. But exercise, including strength training, can help. In one study, women who had breast cancer started a program of either resistance training or cardio exercise during chemotherapy. Both groups saw improvements in their strength, endurance, and quality of life, but the weight lifters had slightly greater gains. And for women suffering from arm swelling after breast cancer surgery (lymphedema), strength training may offer some relief. A study published in *The New England Journal of Medicine* found that those who did weight training twice a week for 13 weeks reported fewer symptoms and flare-ups. The findings call into question the long-held medical view that women who have had breast cancer surgery should avoid stressing the arm for fear that muscle strain could worsen arm swelling.

Lyme disease. Annually, 300,000 Americans are diagnosed with Lyme disease, and over 40% of them have persistent symptoms such as pain, fatigue, and a poor quality of life. But it looks like just a little bit of strength training may have a big impact. Just one set of five exercises done three times a week for four weeks resulted in a sevenfold increase in the number of days people said that they felt healthy and full of energy, according to a small pilot study. More research is needed, but if you have Lyme disease, it might be worth investing in some dumbbells.

Fibromyalgia. This disorder, which is more common in women than men, is characterized by widespread musculoskeletal pain, increased sensitivity to pain, impaired physical abilities, fatigue, and distress. There is currently no cure for fibromyalgia, but exercise, including strength training, appears to offer some hope. A Swedish study of 130 women with fibromyalgia found that those who participated in strength training workouts twice a week for 15 weeks got stronger, reduced their pain by 23%, were better able to deal with their pain, and participated in everyday activities more than the women who didn't exercise. ♦

Should you check with your doctor first?

If you're already doing strength training, you've quite likely taken the necessary precautions. However, if you're new to this type of exercise—or if you're looking to crank up the intensity of your workouts by doing the Medicine Ball Workout (page 34) or Kettlebell Workout (page 38) or adding plyometrics (page 43) to your routine—it's wise to consult with your doctor or physical therapist before starting. That's especially true if you have not been active recently, if you're a smoker or have quit within the past six months, or if you have any injuries or an unstable chronic health condition, including these:

- heart disease (or multiple risk factors for it)
- a respiratory ailment such as asthma
- high blood pressure
- joint or bone disease
- a neurologic illness
- diabetes
- a joint replacement.

Some conditions, such as unstable angina or an abdominal aortic aneurysm (a weak spot in the wall of the body's main artery) can make strength or power training unsafe. Other problems—for example, a joint injury or cataract treatment—may make it unsafe temporarily (see "When exercise is not advisable," page 13); in that case, wait until your doctor gives you the go-ahead. One helpful resource for gauging your ability is the Canadian Society for Exercise Physiologists' updated Physical Activity Readiness Questionnaire (PAR-Q1; www.health.harvard.edu/par-q).

Generally speaking, anyone who is healthy or has a well-controlled health problem, such as high blood pressure or diabetes, can safely do the strength and power training workouts in this report, as long as they start with the Basic Workout or Resistance Band Workout and gradually progress to the more challenging workouts that follow. However, you should stop immediately if you experience certain distress signals from your body (see "Warning signs," at right).

Questions for your doctor

When you ask your doctor whether you should observe any restrictions, it's important to explain exactly what sort of program you hope to undertake. Here are three good questions to ask:

- Do I have any health conditions that would be adversely affected by strength or power training or other types of exercise? (For example, people with poorly controlled high blood pressure generally should avoid isometric exercises, which can raise blood pressure considerably.)
- Will my medications affect exercise in any way or vice versa? (People taking insulin or medicine to lower blood sugar may need to adjust the dose when they exercise, for example.)
- Should I limit the types or intensity of exercises

▶ Warning signs

Never ignore these signs of distress from your body. Stop exercising and call a doctor or 911 right away if you experience any of the following:

- ✔ upper-body discomfort, including chest pain, aching, burning, tightness, or a feeling of uncomfortable fullness
- ✔ wheezing or shortness of breath that takes longer than five minutes to go away
- ✔ faintness or loss of consciousness
- ✔ pain in bones or joints.

These warning signs pertain to any kind of exercise—strength training and aerobic exercise alike.

Persistent or intense muscle pain that starts during a workout or right afterward, or muscle soreness that lasts more than one to two weeks, also merits a call to your doctor. (This is in contrast to normal muscle soreness, which starts 12 to 48 hours after a workout and gradually improves.) You should also call your doctor if the routine you've been doing for a while without discomfort starts to cause you pain.

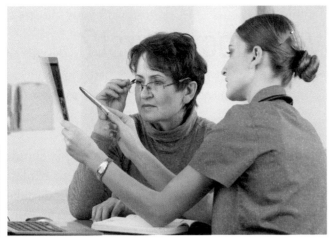

If you have any injuries or an unstable chronic health condition, if you not been active recently, or if you're a smoker, it's wise to check with your doctor before starting strength and power training.

I do? (For example, people who have had a hip replacement may be told to avoid bringing their knees to their chests.)

If you are recovering from certain health problems, your doctor may give you a referral to a physiatrist—a medical doctor who specializes in physical medicine and rehabilitation—or a physical therapist. While physiatrists may tell you what exercises and movements not to do, they generally leave it up to physical therapists to design exercise programs for their patients. Insurance coverage for these services varies, so check with your insurance provider to learn more.

When exercise is not advisable

The National Institute on Aging notes that there are also specific reasons to hold off temporarily on exercise until a doctor advises you that it's safe to resume. These are not specific to strength training; you should not do aerobic exercise, either, if you have any of the following:

- a hernia
- sores on feet or ankles that aren't healing
- hot, swollen joints
- difficulty walking, or lasting pain, after a fall
- blood clots
- a detached or bleeding retina, cataract surgery or a lens implant, or laser eye surgery
- chest pains
- fever (it is usually safe to start exercising again at lighter intensity once the fever has subsided and you feel better)
- irregular, fast, or fluttery heartbeat.

Tips for people with specific conditions

If you have heart disease, diabetes, arthritis, or osteoporosis, it is imperative that you speak with your doctor before you start strength or power training. Once he or she has signed off on your exercise plans, here are some tips that may help you get more out of your workouts and avoid injury.

If you have heart disease

- Be sure to breathe while lifting and lowering weights. Holding your breath while straining can raise blood pressure dangerously. Counting out loud as you exhale may help.
- Be aware that many drugs given to help treat heart disease may affect you when you're exercising. Beta blockers, for example, keep heart rate artificially low; that means your pulse is not a good indicator of how vigorously you are exercising. Vasodilators and ACE inhibitors may make you more prone to dizziness from a drop in blood pressure if your post-exercise cool-down is too short. Talk with your doctor about the medications you take. If you work with an exercise professional, be sure he or she understands the potential effects, too.

If you have diabetes

- Talk with your doctor about adjusting your medications before starting or increasing a strength training program. Exercise, including strength training, uses glucose, so it may affect the dose of medication you need and maybe even the timing of your doses.
- Keep carbohydrates like hard candy or glucose tablets with you when you exercise in case your blood sugar drops precipitously, a condition called hypoglycemia. Signs of hypoglycemia include sweating, trembling, dizziness, hunger, and confusion.
- Wear a diabetes bracelet or ID tag and carry phone numbers in case of emergency while exercising.

If you have arthritis

- Schedule workouts for times of the day when your medications are working well, in order to reduce inflammation and pain. For example, avoid morning workouts if stiffness is at its worst then.

- Before exercise, apply heat to sore joints or take a warm shower or bath. After exercise, cold packs may be helpful.

- If you have rheumatoid arthritis or another form of inflammatory arthritis, include some gentle stretching after you warm up. Inflammation weakens the tendons that tie muscle to bone, making them more susceptible to injury. Remember to use slow movements during your warm-up, and gradually extend your range of motion.

- If you have rheumatoid arthritis, add more rest time to your routine when your condition flares up to reduce inflammation, pain, and fatigue. When it calms down, you can exercise more. Short rest breaks tend to help more than long periods spent in bed.

- Exercise within a comfortable range of motion. If an entire exercise causes significant pain, stop doing it! Discuss other options with your trainer or physical therapist.

- Generally, you should avoid doing strength or power training with actively inflamed joints, at least until the inflammation eases. In some cases, water workouts may be a better choice than strength or power training.

If you have osteoporosis

- Protect your spine. Avoid activities and exercises that require you to bend your spine, especially while lifting a weight.

- Bend your knees when picking up weights to do exercises. You might want to store your weights on a shelf so they are easy to access without injuring your spine.

- Consider trying exercises, such as stair climbing, squats, or lunges, using a weighted vest, especially if you are a postmenopausal woman (see "Buying and using a weighted vest," page 16). Some studies have shown that progressive training using a weighted vest can increase the development of new bone in the hip area and improve balance. ♥

Getting started

W here should strength and power training fit into your exercise plans? What equipment, if any, will you need? This chapter answers those questions and explains the basic terminology used in our strength and power workouts. You will also learn what else a well-rounded exercise program should include in addition to strength and power training.

Buying equipment

The equipment you need for strength and power training depends on the workouts you choose. In this report, there are four different workouts that require different kinds of equipment—dumbbells, resistance bands, a medicine ball, or kettlebells. We recommend that you start with the either the Basic Workout (with dumbbells) or the Resistance Band Workout. Once you've mastered one or both of these, you can choose from one of the other workouts.

Below you'll find descriptions of what you need for each workout. You can buy all of this equipment online. You may also be able to find it at department, discount, or sporting goods stores.

For all the workouts, you should also have a non-slip exercise mat. (A thick carpet will do in a pinch.) The plyometrics exercises require nothing but a good pair of shoes with sturdy support.

For the Basic Workout

- Dumbbells in a few different weights. Depending on your current strength, you might start with as little as a set of 2-pound and 5-pound weights or 5-pound and 8-pound weights. Add heavier weights as needed. Prices start at about $10 for a set and increase for heavier weights. Alternatively, you can buy adjustable dumbbells that offer a variety of weight ranges—for example, from 2.5 to 12.5 pounds or from 5 to 25 pounds. Prices start at about $70 for a set.
- A sturdy chair, preferably without armrests.

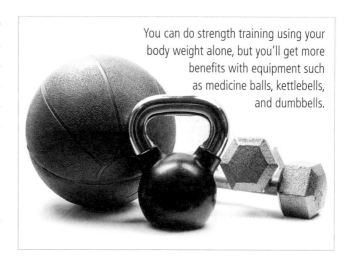

You can do strength training using your body weight alone, but you'll get more benefits with equipment such as medicine balls, kettlebells, and dumbbells.

For the Resistance Band Workout

- Resistance bands or tubes in a variety of resistance levels, designated by color. Bands look like big, wide rubber bands, while the tubes are narrow, have handles, and tend to be more durable. Bands provide more resistance on the eccentric contraction than dumbbells. Prices start at about $10, and many are sold in sets so you get a variety of resistance levels.
- Heavy furniture, poles, or railings to anchor the band for certain moves. In a pinch, you could have someone else hold the band for you. Just make sure that he or she is stronger than you are.

For the Medicine Ball Workout

- Medicine balls, which are about the size of a soccer ball and come in a variety of weights. You can lift or toss them to work your muscles in new ways. Start with a lightweight ball, about 4 to 8 pounds. Some medicine balls bounce, while others don't. You can use either type for the routine in this report. Prices start at about $20.

For the Kettlebell Workout

- Kettlebells, which look like a ball or bell with a handle. Unlike dumbbells, which you grip at the center of the mass, you grip kettlebells outside of their

© mmjimenez I Thinkstock

center of mass. This requires you to exert more muscle force to control the weight, providing a more challenging workout. The lightest kettlebell is usually 5 pounds. Prices start at about $25. Most are sold individually, but some sets are available. There are also adjustable types so you can get multiple weights in one kettlebell.

Optional for all workouts

An optional piece of equipment that you may want to invest in at some point is a weighted vest. A weighted vest can add additional resistance for stationary moves such as bridges and planks. If you use a weighted vest for moving exercises such as lunges or plyometrics, it can help you develop more power. For advice on safe use of a weighted vest, see "Buying and using a weighted vest," below.

Frequently asked questions

The answers to the following questions provide crucial information about strength and power training to ensure that you get a safe and effective workout.

How often should I do strength training?

According to the most recent Physical Activity Guidelines for Americans, issued by the U.S. Department of Health and Human Services, adults ages 18 to 64 should perform a complete strength training routine, about 20 to 30 minutes, two or three times a week. (Of course, once a week is better than not at all, if that's the most you can manage.) Allow at least 48 hours between sessions to let your muscles recover. So, if you do a strength workout on Monday, wait until at least Wednesday to do another one.

The fastest gains are made in the first four to eight weeks; after that, expect progress to slow somewhat.

How often should I do power training?

The Physical Activity Guidelines for Americans do not address power training, but the American College of Sports Medicine (ACSM) has been advocating it for more than five years. Based on research, the ACSM recommends doing power training two or three times

Buying and using a weighted vest

If you want to wear a weighted vest, choose one with removable weights in half-pound to 1-pound bars. The amount of weight you use depends on your body weight. Consult the chart below to determine the maximum amount of weight your vest will need to hold. (The more weight it holds, the more expensive it tends to be.) You can find vests online by searching for "weighted vest," or you may be able to find them at a department store, discount store, or sporting goods store. Prices range from about $30 to more than $200.

Follow the guidelines below to determine how much weight to start with, the amount to add every one to two weeks, and the maximum amount of weight to use. For example, a 150-pound woman would add 3 pounds to her vest every week or two. Over the course of about six to 12 weeks, the weight would increase as follows: 3 pounds, 6 pounds, 9 pounds, 12 pounds, 15 pounds, and finally 18 pounds. She should not put more than 18 pounds into her vest.

If your workout feels too vigorous at any time or if you can't complete the recommended two to three sets of an exercise with the vest on, reduce the amount of weight in your vest to a more comfortable level.

Guidelines for adding weight to your vest

If you weigh	Starting amount of weight; increase the weight in your vest every one to two weeks by this amount	Maximum amount to use in your vest
75–99 pounds	1 pound	7 pounds
100–149 pounds	2 pounds	12 pounds
150–199 pounds	3 pounds	18 pounds
200–239 pounds	4 pounds	20 pounds
240–280 pounds	5 pounds	25 pounds
281–329 pounds	6 pounds	30 pounds
330 pounds or more	7 pounds	35 pounds

a week along with strength training. You can easily do that with the workouts in this report.

Do I still need to do aerobic workouts?

Yes! Aerobic activity is good for better heart health, lower blood pressure, improved diabetes management, sounder sleep, better immune function, sharper mental function, and more. For guidelines on how often to do aerobic exercise, see "What about aerobic exercise?" below.

How much weight or resistance should I use?

Once you understand exactly how to do each exercise, choose a weight (or resistance level for bands) that allows you to do only the recommended number of repetitions (reps). The last one or two reps should be difficult. If you can't lift the weight at least the mini-mum number of reps, use a lighter weight or resistance (see "Training tips," page 19).

If you exercise regularly, your muscles will gradually adapt to the weight you are using so you can do more reps. When you can comfortably perform the maximum number of reps without completely tiring the muscle, it's time to increase the amount of weight.

How quickly (or slowly) should I lift the weights?

The speed, or tempo, at which you perform the exercises will vary depending upon the type of exercise you are doing. Strength training exercises should be done at a 3–1–3 tempo. That means three seconds to lift the weight, one second to hold it in that position, and three seconds to lower the weight. For power training, you'll pick up the pace. You will do the lifting

What about aerobic exercise?

Strength training is only one piece of the exercise puzzle. According to experts, a well-rounded program should also include aerobic activity and flexibility exercises. Here's a summary of what you need.

Aerobic activity. Aerobic activity (also called cardiovascular exercise, or simply cardio) is exercise that speeds heart rate and breathing for sustained periods. Examples include walking, running, cycling, or swimming. According to the Physical Activity Guidelines for Americans from the U.S. Department of Health and Human Services, most adults should aim for at least 150 minutes of moderate aerobic activity a week. Spread your aerobic exercise across the week, so that you are exercising at least three days a week. Each session should last at least 10 minutes.

If you kick up the intensity level of your workouts from moderate to vigorous, you can reduce the total amount of aerobic exercise to 75 minutes a week—or plan an equivalent mix of the two for the appropriate amount of time. (Ten minutes of vigorous activity equals roughly 20 minutes of moderate activity.) According to many exercise guidelines, running is an example of "vigorous" aerobic exercise. "Moderate" exercise might be walking at 3.5 mph. The truth is, though, your level of fitness dictates whether an activity is light, moderate, or vigorous. If you are rarely active, a less-than-brisk walk might qualify as moderate—or even vigorous. Here's a rule of thumb for aerobic exercise: If you can talk easily while performing your routine, exercise harder. If you can't carry on a conversation at all, back off.

Flexibility exercises. Stretch at least twice a week, according to the American College of Sports Medicine (see "Stretching exercises," page 47). Flexibility exercises, or stretches, may expand your range of motion, keep muscles more limber, improve posture and balance, and help prevent falls. Warm muscles are less likely to be injured than cold muscles, so it's best to perform stretches as part of your cool-down following a workout. Or, if you prefer, you can stretch after a five- to 10-minute warm-up, during which you might walk or dance to some songs on the radio. Consider activities such as yoga or tai chi, which help with balance as well as improving flexibility.

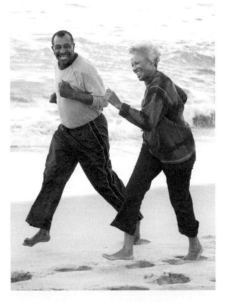

A sedentary lifestyle is one of the major risk factors for heart disease. Regular physical activity—such as walking, gardening, or golfing—can reduce your risks.

as quickly as possible while maintaining good form. The rest of the exercise is performed at the slower tempo used for strength training: You hold at the top of the move for one second, then take three seconds to lower. (See "Tempo" on page 22 for more directions.)

How many sets of each exercise should I do?

Strength training aims to tire the muscles that are being worked. According to numerous scientific reviews, the best way to do this is to perform three sets of each exercise. (A set consists of a recommended number of reps.) That doesn't mean you should skip a workout if you have time for only one set—you get the most strength and toning benefits from the first set, especially if you're a beginner, with subsequent sets providing diminishing returns. However, the more you train, the more important it will be to do three sets in order to achieve the best results and continue gaining strength.

How long should I rest between sets?

Resting for one to three minutes between sets nets the best strength gains. The higher the intensity of your workout (meaning the heavier the weights you're lifting), the more rest you'll need. For most people, a minute or two is ample. During this time, your body generates hormonal and metabolic responses that build and strengthen muscles. In addition, resting enables your muscles to perform better on your next set. If you don't rest at all, your muscles may be too tired for you to lift with good form, increasing your risk of injury. Conversely, resting too long may also be risky, because your muscles cool down, making them more susceptible to injury.

Do I need to hire a trainer or join a gym?

No one needs to join a gym to exercise regularly. Your body offers the cheapest equipment available, and spending a little money on basic equipment like dumbbells or resistance bands can deliver great gains. At home, you needn't worry about how you look to others or whether you'll have time to make it to the gym. And the sums saved by not paying for a gym might be put to good use elsewhere, whether that means monthly bills or tennis lessons.

But joining a gym may be a good move for some people. Spending money on a gym membership may motivate you to get your money's worth. For others, classes offer companionship and a safe way to learn technique (provided that the classes are geared to your ability level). And the wide range of equipment and classes provide variety to keep you challenged and interested in working out.

Before deciding whether a gym is right for you, consider your preferences and needs. Ask yourself some questions: How far must you travel to the gym, and are you likely to make the trek? Do the gym's hours of operation work well for you? Consider what amenities you are likely to use—classes, trainers, or just equipment—and don't pay for ones you won't use.

Do I need a trainer?

While you can certainly follow our workouts on your own, trainers have valuable skills to tap. They can teach you to work out safely and maintain good form, introduce you to new equipment, and update an exercise program to keep you motivated. They also might push you to work harder than you would on your own. And they can tailor an exercise program to any goals you choose: enhancing health and appearance, losing weight, charging through a triathlon, or another aim entirely.

No nationwide licensing requirements exist for personal trainers. So in addition to seeking a good match in personalities and respect for your goals, you should ask about these points:

Certification. Certifying organizations include the American College of Sports Medicine (ACSM), American Council on Exercise (ACE), National Academy of Sports Medicine (NASM), and other groups whose certifications are recognized by the National Commission for Certifying Agencies (NCCA).

Experience. Years of experience matter, as does experience in working with others like you, whether you're a gifted athlete or a confirmed sloth with tricky knees. Some trainers specialize in working with particular populations—older adults, athletes, pregnant women, cancer survivors—and may have taken courses and possibly certifying exams in these areas.

References. Ask health care providers such as doctors, physical therapists, chiropractors, massage therapists, dietitians, and friends for referrals. Certifying organizations like ACE and ACSM often have referral systems. Before signing on with a trainer, ask for references and call a few.

Liability insurance. Whether a trainer works for a gym or independently, make sure he or she has liability insurance.

Training tips

The following guidelines apply to any strength training program you choose.

- Drink plenty of water throughout the day and whenever you exercise in order to prevent headaches and fatigue.

- Never sacrifice proper form and good posture for the sake of lifting heavier weights or going faster. It's easiest to learn good form through a class or one-on-one sessions with a well-trained exercise professional. If that's not possible, exercise in front of a mirror so you can check your form (see "Posture and alignment: Striking the right pose," below).

- Breathe out as you lift or exert force; breathe in as you lower or release. Don't hold your breath, as this can cause your blood pressure to rise. Counting out loud as you lift will prevent you from holding your breath.

- Focus on the muscles you are working. In a recent study from Denmark, participants increased muscle activity up to 35% when they thought about the muscles they were working as they performed the exercise. The more muscle activity, the more results you'll get.

- Isolate muscles by trying to move only the muscles you're exercising. This will prevent other muscles from helping out and minimizing the strengthening benefits to the muscles you're trying to work. Don't rock or sway.

- Lift or push and release weights smoothly, without jerking. Jerky movements can sometimes lead to spraining or straining a muscle, tendon, or ligament.

- Don't lock your joints; always leave a slight bend in your knees and elbows when straightening out your legs and arms. Hyperextended joints can strain ligaments around the joint. This is especially important when doing jumping exercises like those in "Bonus power moves: Plyometrics" (see page 43).

- When moving your arms or legs, stick with a range that feels comfortable. These exercises should not cause pain while you are doing them. Over time, gradually extend your range of motion through exercise and stretching.

- Listen to your body, and cut back if you aren't able to finish a series of exercises or an exercise session, can't talk while exercising, feel faint after a session, feel tired during the day, or suffer joint aches and pains after a session.

- Build up slowly over time. Don't be so eager to see results that you risk hurting yourself by exercising too long or too often or by choosing too much weight. Remember that it's important to rest muscles for at least 48 hours between sessions.

- If you injure yourself, remember RICE (rest, ice, compression, and elevation). Rest the injured muscle. Ice it for 20 to 30 minutes every two to three hours during the first two or three days. Apply compression with an elastic bandage whenever you're out of bed until the swelling resolves. Elevate the injured area while resting or icing. Call your doctor for advice and information about managing pain or swelling. Wait until the injury heals before doing strength training on that muscle again, and start with a lower weight.

If you don't want to wait one to three minutes, cutting rest time between sets to 30 seconds keeps your heart rate and calorie burn up, so you reap some aerobic and weight-loss benefits during a strength training session. It's wise to note, however, that this lessens strength and muscle gains. It's a trade-off that each person should evaluate. If you do choose to cut your rest time, adjust the amount of weight you are lifting to be sure you don't sacrifice good form.

Posture and alignment: Striking the right pose

Exercise is important, but if you don't do it right, you run the risk of injuring yourself. You will also slow gains because you aren't isolating muscles properly.

Posture helps more than you might think. In fact, good posture and alignment help anytime you're moving. For example, if you bend at your waist while doing arm curls or the overhead press (see page 26 for both exercises), this puts stress on your lower back that may result in an injury. And changing the posture or alignment of an exercise can change the muscles that are being worked. For example, if you keep your elbows in close to your body during a push-up, you will work your triceps (the backs of your arms) more than your chest muscles. Depending upon the routine you are doing, that may be fine. For our routine, the kneeling push-up (page 24) should target your chest muscles more, so the description tells you to point your elbows out to the sides. That's why it's important to read and follow the instructions carefully.

The exercises in our workouts often call for you to stand up straight. That means

- your chin is parallel to the floor
- both shoulders are back and down
- both wrists are firm and straight, not flexed upward or downward
- both hips are even
- both knees are pointed straight ahead
- both feet are pointed straight ahead
- body weight is distributed evenly on both feet.

In addition, it's important to maintain a neutral spine. A neutral spine takes into account the slight natural curves of the spine, but it's not flexed or arched. One way to find the neutral position is to lift your tailbone as far as comfortable to arch your lower back, then tuck your tailbone under to flatten your lower back. The spot approximately in the middle should be neutral. If you're not used to standing or sitting up straight, it may take a while for this to feel natural. When you are instructed to bend, do so at the hips, not at the waist, and keep your spine neutral and your core muscles contracted to protect your back.

Few of us have perfect posture, which is why it's so important to check your posture before and during each exercise. Each exercise in our workouts offers tips on good technique, so make sure you review them before trying the move. Looking in a mirror as you do exercises helps enormously. It enables you to observe your body position and correct sloppy form.

Paying attention as you perform upper-body exercises may also alert you to muscle imbalances based on whether your right or left side is dominant. If you notice this, focus on your weaker side to make sure it's not slacking off. Over time, this will help to even out the imbalance and give you a better workout.

The workouts

This report includes four strength and power workouts that use different types of equipment—dumbbells, resistance bands, a medicine ball, and a kettlebell. In addition, there are plyometrics (jumping exercises) that you can add to any of the workouts once you've progressed through the other routines.

If you are new to strength training or have not been doing it regularly for the past month, we recommend that you start with the strength version of either the Basic Workout (page 23) or the Resistance Band Workout (page 28). For at least two to four weeks, follow the "strength" instructions for reps and tempo. These routines will help you build a strong foundation.

When you feel comfortable with these, you can turn either of the routines into a power workout by following the "power" instructions for reps and tempo. Or you can advance to one of the other two workouts—the Medicine Ball Workout (page 34) or the Kettlebell Workout (page 38)—which incorporate both strength and power training. Give yourself another two to four weeks, and then you can add some high-impact, power-boosting plyometrics (page 43) to your workouts, if you desire.

Don't forget to warm up before you begin, and cool down afterward. Then, spend a few minutes doing the stretching exercises (page 47) to complete your workout.

Always remember to maintain good posture and alignment (see page 19) and follow our training tips (page 19) to minimize your risk of injury.

Warm-up

Before doing any of the workouts, spend five to 10 minutes warming up all major muscle groups. A warm-up enables your body to ease into exercise so you'll feel better. Your heart rate and breathing gradually increase, pumping more nutrient-rich, oxygenated blood to your muscles for exercise. Your joints become more lubricated and your muscles more pliable so they perform better, and you're less susceptible to discomfort or even an injury.

Excellent ways to warm up include marching in place and gently swinging your arms, walking on a treadmill, pedaling an exercise bike, or mimicking the workout exercises without holding any weights. Start slowly, and gradually increase your pace. (Stretching is no longer recommended as a warm-up, unless it's a "dynamic" stretch that involves movement; to see a short routine, go to www.health.harvard.edu/dynamic-stretches.)

Cool-down

Cooling down slows breathing and heartbeat, gradually routing blood back into its normal circulatory patterns. This helps prevent a sudden drop in blood pressure that can cause dizziness, especially if you bend over or straighten up quickly (a reaction called postural hypotension). After your workout, spend five to 10 minutes cooling down by walking around. The more intense your workout and the higher your heart rate, the longer your cool-down should be. Don't forget to stretch afterward (see "Stretching exercises," page 47).

Key to the instructions

Each of the exercises in our workouts includes certain directions—including your starting position and the movement you will make during each exercise—along with tips and techniques to help. We also use certain terms you'll need to know.

Repetitions (reps). Each time you perform the movement in an exercise, that's called a rep. If you cannot do all the reps at first, just do what you can, and then gradually increase reps as you improve. When you are training for strength, aim for eight to 12 reps. For power training, you'll do fewer reps—six to 10—but at a faster pace (see "Tempo," below).

Set. One set is a specific number of repetitions. For example, eight to 12 reps often make a single set. Usually, we suggest doing one to three sets.

Tempo. This tells you the count for the key movements in an exercise. For example, 3–1–3 means lift a weight in three counts, hold for one count, then lower it on a count of three. Exercises with more parts have more numbers, and some, like the halo (page 39), have only one number, meaning the exercise is one fluid movement.

Hold. While most exercises have a hold as part of the tempo, the stretching exercises list "Hold" as a separate line, since that is the focus of stretches. It tells you the number of seconds to hold each stretch.

Rest. Resting gives your muscles a chance to recharge and helps you maintain good form. Except during the warm-up and cool-down activities, we specify a range of time to rest between sets. How much of this time you need will differ depending on your level of fitness and how heavy your weights are. (See "How long should I rest between sets?" on page 18.)

In addition, each set of instructions offers options to "make it easier" or "make it harder." These variations modify the exercise to be less challenging (for beginners or those with health concerns) or to increase the difficulty (for more advanced exercisers). ▼

Basic Workout

The Basic Workout is good for everyone. If you're new to strength training—or haven't been exercising for a month or more—this dumbbell and bodyweight routine is a great starting point. But even if you lift weights regularly, this workout can help by targeting muscles in new ways. As you grow stronger, you can continue to challenge yourself with this routine by using heavier weights, by doing the "make it harder" variations for each exercise, or by turning the strength workout into a power routine.

To convert the strength routine into a power workout: Simply change the tempos of the exercises. Each exercise lists two different tempos—the slower one for strength and the faster one for power. For example, in the bent-over row (page 25), instead of lifting on a count of 3, holding for 1, and lowering for another 3, you would start by lifting on a count of just 1, then holding for 1, and lowering for 3. (To see an example illustrating the difference, go to the video at www.health.harvard.edu/strength-to-power.)

If you're a beginner: You should follow the instructions for the standard, strength form of each exercise for at least two weeks before moving on to the power variations or the "make it harder" options. That way, you will become familiar with the exercises and build a base of strength to avoid injury as you progress. You should also do at least two weeks of power training before moving on to the more advanced Medicine Ball Workout (page 34) or Kettlebell Workout (page 38), which incorporate both strength and power training.

For variety, you can alternate the Basic Workout with the Resistance Band Workout (page 28), which is another good routine for beginners.

---

① Reverse lunge

Muscles worked: Gluteus, quadriceps, hamstrings, gastrocnemius, erector spinae

Reps: 8–12 for strength, 6–10 for power
Sets: 1–3
Tempo: 3–1–3 for strength,
3–1–1 for power
Rest: 30–90 seconds between sets

Starting position: Stand up straight with your feet together and your arms at your sides, holding dumbbells.

Movement: Step back onto the ball of your left foot, bend your knees, and lower into a lunge. Your right knee should align over your right ankle, and your left knee should point toward the floor. Push off your back foot to stand up and return to the starting position. Repeat, stepping back with your right foot to do the lunge on the opposite side. This is one rep.

Tips and techniques:
- Keep your spine neutral when lowering into the lunge.
- Don't lean forward.
- As you bend your knees, lower the back knee directly down to the floor with the thigh perpendicular to the floor.

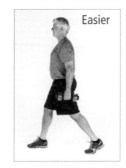
Easier

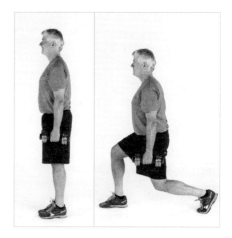

◄ **Make it easier:** Do stationary lunges, so that you're not stepping back with one foot at the beginning of each lunge. Simply stand with one foot in front of the other and bend your knees. Finish all reps, then switch legs and repeat to complete one set. Or, do lunges without weights.

Make it harder: Step forward into the lunges, or use heavier weights.

The editors would like to thank Philip L. Penny and Michele Stanten for serving as models for the workouts.

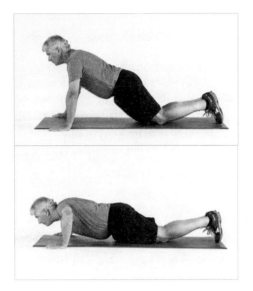

② Kneeling push-up

Muscles worked: Pectoralis, deltoids, triceps, rectus abdominis, erector spinae, gluteus

Reps: 8–12 for strength,
 6–10 for power
Sets: 1–3
Tempo: 3–1–3 for strength,
 3–1–1 for power
Rest: 30–90 seconds between sets

Starting position: Begin on the floor on all fours with your hands slightly more than shoulder-width apart. Walk your hands forward and lower your hips so your body is at a 45-degree angle to the floor and forms a straight line from head to knees.

Movement: Bend your elbows out to the sides and slowly lower your upper body toward the floor until your elbows are bent about 90 degrees. Press against the floor and straighten your arms to return to the starting position.

Tips and techniques:
• Keep your head in line with your spine.
• Keep your abs tight to prevent your back from arching too much.

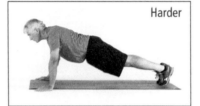

Harder

Make it easier: Stand up and do push-ups with your hands against a wall or a countertop.

◄ **Make it harder:** Lift your knees off the floor and do push-ups balancing on your hands and your toes and balls of your feet.

---

③ Wood chop

Muscles worked: Pectoralis, deltoids, gluteus, obliques, quadriceps, hamstrings, erector spinae

Reps: 8–12 on each side for strength,
 6–10 on each side for power
Sets: 1–3
Tempo: 3–1–3 for strength,
 1–1–3 for power
Rest: 30–90 seconds between sets

Starting position: Stand with your feet about shoulder-width apart and hold a dumbbell with both hands. Hinge forward at your hips and bend your knees to sit back into a squat. Rotate your torso to the right and extend your arms to hold the dumbbell on the outside of your right knee.

Movement: Straighten your legs to stand up as you rotate your torso to the left and raise the weight diagonally across your body and up to the left just above your left shoulder. Keep your arms extended. In a chopping motion, slowly bring the medicine ball down and across your body toward the outside of your right knee. This is one rep. Finish all reps, then repeat on the other side. This completes one set.

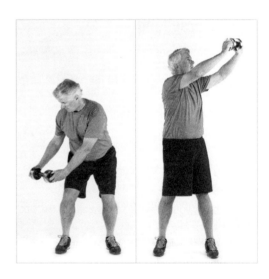

Tips and techniques:
• Keep your spine neutral and your shoulders down and back.
• Reach only as far as is comfortable.
• Keep your knees behind your toes when you squat.

Make it easier: Do the exercise without a dumbbell.

Make it harder: Use a heavier dumbbell.

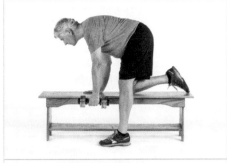

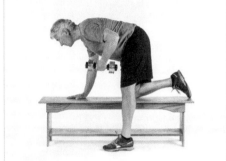

(4) Bent-over row

Muscles worked: Latissimus dorsi, trapezius, rhomboids, deltoids, biceps

Reps: 8–12 with each arm for strength, 6–10 with each arm for power
Sets: 1–3
Tempo: 3–1–3 for strength, 1–1–3 for power
Rest: 30–90 seconds between sets

Starting position: Stand with a weight in your left hand and a bench or sturdy chair at your right side. Place your right hand and knee on the bench or chair seat. Let your left arm hang directly under your right shoulder, fully extended toward the floor. Your spine should be neutral and your shoulders and hips squared.

Movement: Squeeze your shoulder blades together, then bend your elbow to slowly lift the weight toward your ribs. Return to the starting position. Finish all reps, then repeat with the opposite arm. This completes one set.

Tips and techniques:
• Keep your shoulders squared throughout.
• Keep your elbow close to your side as you lift the weight.
• Keep your head in line with your spine.

Make it easier: Use a lighter weight.
Make it harder: Use a heavier weight.

---

(5) Bridge

Muscles worked: Gluteus, hamstrings, erector spinae

Reps: 8–12 for strength, 6–10 for power
Sets: 1–3
Tempo: 3–1–3 for strength, 1–1–3 for power
Rest: 30–90 seconds between sets

Starting position: Lie on your back with your knees bent and feet flat on the floor, hip-width apart. Place your arms at your sides, palms up. Relax your shoulders against the floor.

Movement: Tighten your buttocks, then lift your hips up off the floor as high as is comfortable. Keep your hips even and spine neutral. Return to the starting position.

Tips and techniques:
• Don't press your hands or arms against the floor to help you lift.
• Keep your shoulders, hips, knees, and feet evenly aligned.
• Keep your shoulders down and relaxed against the floor.

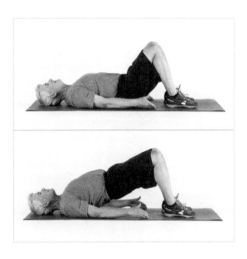

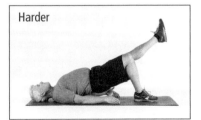

Harder

Make it easier: Lift your buttocks just slightly off the floor.

◄ **Make it harder:** Extend one leg off the floor to do one-leg bridges.

QUICK BASIC WORKOUT

On days when you feel that you just don't have time for a full workout, do this abbreviated routine. Some exercise is better than none!

• **Kneeling push-up** (page 24)
• **Wood chop** (page 24)
• **Bent-over row** (above)
• **Superman** (page 26)

⑥ Superman

Muscles worked: Deltoids, latissimus dorsi, erector spinae, gluteus, hamstrings

Reps: 8–12 for strength, 6–10 for power
Sets: 1–3
Tempo: 3–1–3 for strength, 1–1–3 for power
Rest: 30–90 seconds between sets

Starting position: Lie facedown on the floor with your arms extended, palms down, and your legs extended.

Movement: Simultaneously lift your arms, head, chest, and legs up off the floor as high as is comfortable. Hold. Return to the starting position.

Tips and techniques:
• Tighten your buttocks before lifting.
• Don't look up.
• Keep your shoulders down, away from your ears.

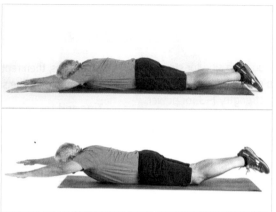

Make it easier: Lift your right arm and left leg while keeping the opposite arm and leg on the floor. Switch sides with each rep.

Make it harder: Hold in the "up" position for three to five seconds before lowering.

⑦ Overhead press

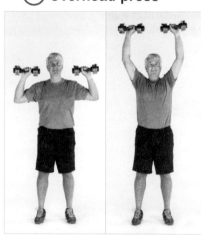

Muscles worked:
Deltoids, triceps

Reps: 8–12 for strength, 6–10 for power
Sets: 1–3
Tempo: 3–1–3 for strength, 1–1–3 for power
Rest: 30–90 seconds between sets

Starting position: Stand tall with your feet about shoulder-width apart, your chest lifted, and shoulders back and down. Hold a dumbbell in each hand at shoulder height with your palms facing forward and elbows pointing out to the sides.

Movement: Slowly raise the weights straight up until your arms are fully extended. Hold. Slowly lower the dumbbells back to the starting position.

Tips and techniques:
• Keep your abs tight.
• Keep your spine neutral and your shoulders down and back.
• Don't pull your elbows back in starting position.

Make it easier: Sit on a chair.
Make it harder: Use heavier weights.

⑧ Arm curls

Muscles worked:
Biceps

Reps: 8–12 for strength, 6–10 for power
Sets: 1–3
Tempo: 3–1–3 for strength, 1–1–3 for power
Rest: 30–90 seconds between sets

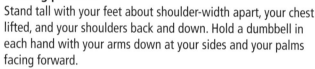

Starting position:
Stand tall with your feet about shoulder-width apart, your chest lifted, and your shoulders back and down. Hold a dumbbell in each hand with your arms down at your sides and your palms facing forward.

Movement: Slowly bend your elbows, lifting the dumbbells toward your shoulders. Hold. Slowly lower the dumbbells, straightening your arms back to the starting position.

Tips and techniques:
• Keep your abs tight.
• Keep your spine neutral and your shoulders down and back.
• Keep your upper arm still and your elbows close to your sides.

Make it easier: Sit in a chair, or use lighter weights.
Make it harder: Use heavier weights.

⑨ Side plank

Muscles worked: Erector spinae, rectus abdominis, obliques, transverse abdominis

Reps: 2–4 on each side for strength, 6–10 on each side for power
Sets: 1 for strength, 1–3 for power
Tempo: Hold the plank position 15–60 seconds for strength; use tempo of 1–1–3 for power
Rest: 30–90 seconds between reps (for strength) or sets (for power)

Starting position: Lie in a straight line on your right side. Support your upper body on your right forearm with your shoulder aligned directly over your elbow. Stack your left foot on top of your right foot. Rest your left hand on your side.

Movement: Tighten your abdominal muscles. Exhale as you lift your right hip and right leg off the floor and raise your left arm toward the ceiling. Keeping shoulders and hips in a straight line, balance on your right forearm and the side of your right foot. Hold. Return to the starting position. This is one rep. Fin-

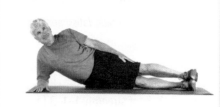
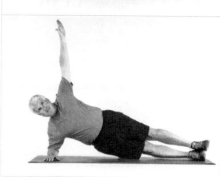

ish all reps, then repeat on your left side. This completes one set.

Tips and techniques:
• Keep your head and spine neutral, and align your shoulder over your elbow.
• Focus on lifting the bottom hip.
• Keep your shoulders down and back.

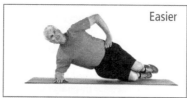
Easier

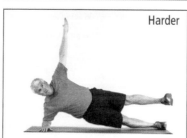
Harder

◄ **Make it easier:** Bend at your knees and put your feet behind you. Keep your knees and lower legs on the floor as you lift your hips.

◄ **Make it harder:** Lift your top foot up as you hold.

⑩ Reverse fly

Muscles worked: Deltoids, rhomboids, trapezius

Reps: 8–12 for strength, 6–10 for power
Sets: 1–3
Tempo: 3–1–3 for strength, 1–1–3 for power
Rest: 30–90 seconds between sets

Starting position: Sit on the edge of a chair, holding a weight in each hand. Hinge forward at your hips, bringing your chest toward your thighs and keeping your back in a straight line. Your arms should hang next to your calves with your palms facing toward your body and thumbs pointing forward.

Movement: Squeeze your shoulder blades together, then slowly lift the weights out to the sides until your arms are at about shoulder height. Keep your elbows soft, not locked. Pause, then return to the starting position.

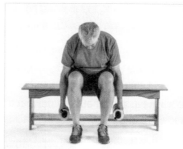
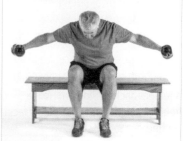

Tips and techniques:
• Throughout the movement, squeeze your shoulder blades together.
• Control the movement without using any momentum.
• Exhale as you lift.

Make it easier: Use lighter weights or no weights.
Make it harder: Use heavier weights. ♥

Resistance Band Workout

Here is another routine that is good for all levels. And since resistance bands are lightweight and packable, they are a great option for anyone who travels a lot. That means there's no excuse for missing a strength workout when you're on the road. Bands also target some muscles such as the latissimus dorsi that are harder to work with dumbbells. In addition, they place more consistent tension on the muscles throughout the range of motion. With dumbbells, the tension varies. Both are beneficial, which is why it's good to mix up your routine.

If you're a beginner: Follow the instructions for the standard form of each exercise for at least two weeks before moving on to the power versions or the "make it harder" variations. This will allow you to become familiar with the exercises and build a base of strength to avoid injury as you progress.

If you have experience in strength training: You can use bands that offer greater resistance. If that's not hard enough, you can hold dumbbells (start with light weights) as you do the band exercises to get a really challenging workout that offers the best of both pieces of equipment.

Everyone should do at least two weeks of power training (beginners may want to do more) before moving on to the more advanced Medicine Ball Workout (page 34) and Kettlebell Workout (page 38), which incorporate both strength and power training. You can alternate this routine with the Basic Workout (page 23) for variety.

① Upright row

Muscles worked: Deltoids, trapezius, biceps

Reps: 8–12 for strength,
   6–10 for power
Sets: 1–3
Tempo: 3–1–3 for strength,
   1–1–3 for power
Rest: 30–90 seconds between sets

Starting position: Place the band under both feet. Grasp each end of the band with your palms up. Then flip your hands over so your palms are facing you and the ends of the band hang inside your hands toward each other. Stand tall with your arms extending down in front of you.

Movement: Bend your elbows out to the sides and pull the band to chest height. Hold. Slowly extend your arms and return to the starting position, resisting the pull of the band.

Tips and techniques:
- Don't arch your back, and keep your abs tight.
- Keep your shoulders down and back, away from your ears.
- Keep your wrists straight, in line with your arms.

▶ **Make it easier:** Stand on the band with only one foot so there is more slack in the band. Alternatively, you can place your hands closer to the ends of the band for less resistance, or use a lighter resistance band.

Make it harder: Place your hands closer to the center of the band for more resistance, or use a heavier resistance band.

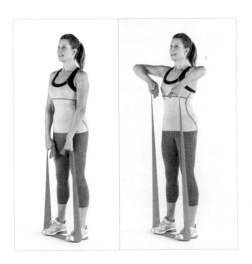

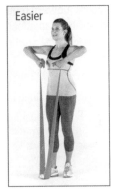

Easier

② Chest press

Muscles worked: Pectoralis, deltoids, triceps

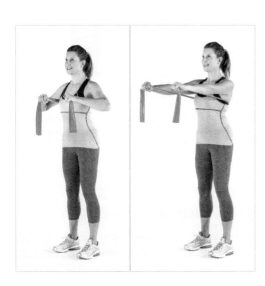

Reps: 8–12 for strength,
6–10 for power
Sets: 1–3
Tempo: 3–1–3 for strength,
1–1–3 for power
Rest: 30–90 seconds between sets

Starting position: Stand tall with your feet about shoulder-width apart. Place a band around your back and under your arms. Hold each end with your arms bent, elbows pointing out and your hands by your armpits.

Movement: Extend your arms straight out in front of you at chest height, stretching the band. Slowly bend your arms and return to the starting position, resisting the pull of the band.

Tips and techniques:
• Don't arch your back, and keep your abs tight.
• Keep your shoulders down and back, away from your ears.
• Keep your wrists straight, in line with your arms.

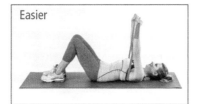

Easier

◄ **Make it easier:** Place your hands closer to the ends of the band for less resistance, or use a lighter resistance band. You can also do this move lying faceup on the floor with your legs bent.

Make it harder: Place your hands closer to the center of the band for more resistance, or use a heavier resistance band.

③ Pull-down

Muscles worked: Latissimus dorsi, biceps

Reps: 8–12 for strength,
6–10 for power
Sets: 1–3
Tempo: 3–1–3 for strength,
1–1–3 for power
Rest: 30–90 seconds between sets

Starting position: Stand tall with your feet about shoulder-width apart. Hold a band overhead with your arms extended and your hands about 12 to 18 inches apart.

Movement: Bend your elbows and pull your hands down, stretching the band, to about shoulder level. Slowly raise your arms back overhead to the starting position, resisting the pull of the band.

Tips and techniques:
• Don't arch your back, and keep your abs tight.
• Keep your shoulders down and back, away from your ears.
• Keep your wrists straight, in line with your arms.

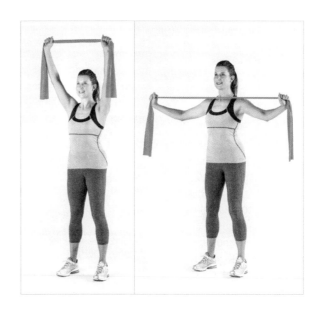

Make it easier: Place your hands closer to the ends of the band for less resistance, or use a lighter resistance band.

Make it harder: Place your hands closer to the center of the band for more resistance, or use a heavier resistance band.

④ Seated row with rotation

Muscles worked: Rhomboids, latissimus dorsi, biceps, obliques

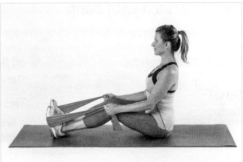
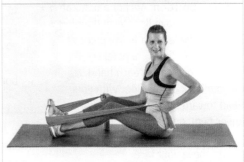

Reps: 8–12 for strength,
6–10 for power
Sets: 1–3
Tempo: 3–1–3 for strength,
1–1–3 for power
Rest: 30–90 seconds between sets

Starting position: Sit on the floor with your legs bent slightly and the band wrapped around the arches of your feet. Grasp each end of the band with your arms extended, palms facing each other.

Movement: Bend your left elbow and pull the band toward your rib cage, keeping your left elbow close to your body and pointing behind you. As you pull, slowly rotate your torso to the left. Hold. Slowly extend your arm and return to the starting posi-tion, resisting the pull of the band. Repeat with your right arm. This is one rep.

Tips and techniques:
• Don't lean back as you pull the band.
• Keep your shoulders down and back, away from your ears.
• Keep your wrists straight, in line with your arms.

Make it easier: Place your hands closer to the ends of the band for less resistance, or use a lighter resistance band. You can also do the seated row without the rotation.

Make it harder: Place your hands closer to the center of the band for more resistance, or use a heavier resistance band.

⑤ Leg press

Muscles worked: Quadriceps

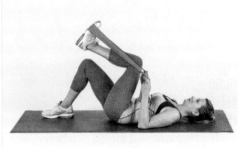
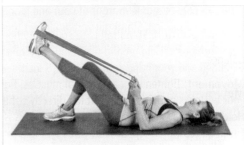

Reps: 8–12 with each leg for strength, 6–10 with each leg for power
Sets: 1–3
Tempo: 3–1–3 for strength,
1–1–3 for power
Rest: 30–90 seconds between sets

Starting position: Lie on your back on the floor with your knees bent and feet flat on the floor. Raise your left foot off the floor, bringing your knee toward your chest. Loop the band around the arch of your foot and hold an end of the band in each hand with your hands by your knee.

Movement: Extend your leg, press-ing your foot away from you. Slowly return to the starting position. This is one rep. Finish all reps, then repeat with your right leg. This completes one set.

Tips and techniques:
• Don't lock your knee as you straighten your leg.
• Extend your leg out on a diagonal, not up toward the ceiling.
• Keep your abs tight.

Make it easier: Place your hands closer to the ends of the band for less resistance, or use a lighter resistance band.

Make it harder: Place your hands closer to the center of the band for more resistance, or use a heavier resistance band.

⑥ Ab crunch with band

Muscles worked: Rectus abdominis, transverse abdominis, psoas major

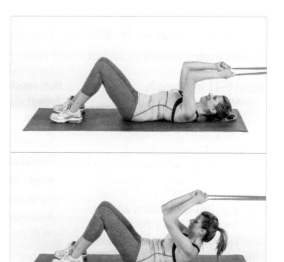

Reps: 8–12 for strength,
6–10 for power
Sets: 1–3
Tempo: 3–1–3 for strength,
1–1–3 for power
Rest: 30–90 seconds between sets

Starting position: Anchor a band at a foot or so above floor level (looping it around the leg of a heavy piece of furniture, a railing, or a pole) so you can grasp one end in each hand. Lie on your back on the floor with your head toward the anchor point, your knees bent, and your feet flat on the floor. Bend your arms and position your hands above your face.

Movement: Contract your abs and lift your head, shoulders, and upper body off the floor. Slowly lower to the starting position.

Tips and techniques:

• Keep your head in line with your spine. Don't point your chin up to the ceiling or down to your chest.

• Exhale as you lift and inhale as you lower.

• Keep your abs tight and tail-bone tucked under.

Make it easier: Move closer to the anchor point or adjust your hand position on the band so it has more slack for less resistance, use a lighter resistance band, or do the exercise without a band.

Make it harder: Move farther away from the anchor point or choke up on the band for more resistance, or use a heavier resistance band.

---

⑦ Hip extension

Muscles worked: Gluteus

Reps: 8–12 with each leg for strength,
6–10 with each leg for power
Sets: 1–3
Tempo: 3–1–3 for strength, 1–1–3 for power
Rest: 30–90 seconds between sets

Starting position: Anchor a band at a foot or so above floor level (tie it around the leg of a heavy piece of furniture, a railing, or a pole in front of you) and loop the band around your left leg. Stand tall with your feet together. You can lightly hold on to the back of chair if needed for balance.

Movement: Tighten your abdominal muscles. Tighten your buttocks and raise your left leg directly behind you. Hold. Slowly lower to the starting position. This is one rep. Finish all reps, then repeat with your right leg. This completes one set.

Tips and techniques:

• Keep your hips even and maintain neutral posture.

• Raise your leg directly behind you, not angled out to the side.

• Remain upright as you lift; don't lean your torso forward.

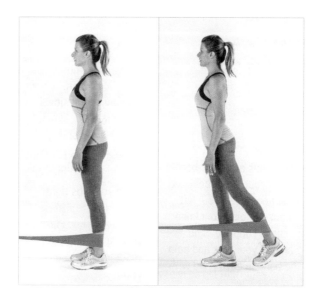

Make it easier: Move closer to the anchor point so the band has more slack for less resistance, use a lighter resistance band, or do the exercise without a band.

Make it harder: Move farther away from the anchor point for more resistance, or use a heavier resistance band.

(8) Soccer kick

Muscles worked: Adductors

Reps: 8–12 with each leg for strength, 6–10 with each leg for power

Sets: 1–3

Tempo: 3–1–3 for strength, 1–1–3 for power

Rest: 30–90 seconds between sets

Starting position: Anchor a band near floor level (tie it around the leg of a heavy piece of furniture, a railing, or a pole) and loop it around your left leg. Stand tall with the anchor point on your left and your left foot out to the side. You can lightly hold on to the back of chair with your left hand if needed for balance.

Movement: Tighten your abdominal muscles. Point your left foot out to the left side, then lift your foot and slowly sweep it diagonally in front of you as if kicking a soccer ball with the inside of your foot. Flex your foot as you swing it. Hold. Slowly bring your foot back to the left side. This is one rep. Finish all reps, then turn around to repeat with the right leg. This completes one set.

Tips and techniques:

• Keep your hips even and maintain neutral posture throughout.

• Tighten your abdominal muscles and the buttock of the standing leg.

• Don't twist your body as you kick.

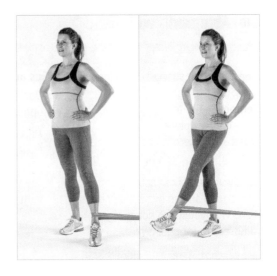

Make it easier: Move closer to the anchor point so the band has more slack for less resistance, use a lighter resistance band, or do the exercise without a band.

Make it harder: Move farther away from the anchor point for more resistance, or use a heavier resistance band.

(9) Side leg lift

Muscles worked: Abductors

Reps: 8–12 with each leg for strength, 6–10 with each leg for power

Sets: 1–3

Tempo: 3–1–3 for strength, 1–1–3 for power

Rest: 30–90 seconds between sets

Starting position: Anchor a band near floor level (tie it around the leg of a heavy piece of furniture, a railing, or a pole) and stand with the anchor point on your left. Loop the band around your right leg so it passes in front of your left leg. Stand tall with your feet together and your hands on your hips. You can lightly hold on to the back of chair if needed for balance.

Movement: Tighten your abdominal muscles. Slowly raise your right foot out to your right side. Flex your foot as you lift. Hold. Slowly lower back to the starting position. This is one rep. Finish all reps, then turn around to repeat with your left leg. This completes one set.

Tips and techniques:

• Keep your hips even and maintain neutral posture throughout.

• Tighten your abdominal muscles and the buttock of the standing leg.

• Don't lean to the side as you lift.

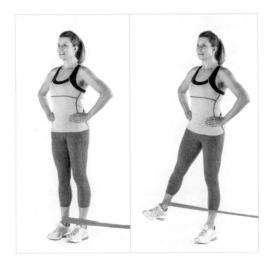

Make it easier: Move closer to the anchor point so the band has more slack for less resistance, use a lighter resistance band, or do the exercise without a band.

Make it harder: Move farther away from the anchor point for more resistance, or use a heavier resistance band.

⑩ Arm curl

Muscles worked: Biceps

Reps: 8–12 for strength, 6–10 for power
Sets: 1–3
Tempo: 3–1–3 for strength,
  1–1–3 for power
Rest: 30–90 seconds between sets

Starting position: Stand on the band, with your feet about shoulder width apart. Hold an end of the band in each hand with your arms down at your sides, palms facing forward.

Movement: Bend your elbows and raise your hands toward your shoulders. Keep your upper arms stationary and your elbows close to your body. Slowly lower to the starting position.

Tips and techniques:
• Don't move your shoulders or upper arms. The movement is at your elbows.
• Keep your shoulders down and back, away from your ears.
• Keep your wrists straight, in line with your arms.

Make it easier: Place the band under only one foot for more slack and for less resistance.

Make it harder: Place your hands closer to the center of the band for more resistance, or use a heavier resistance band.

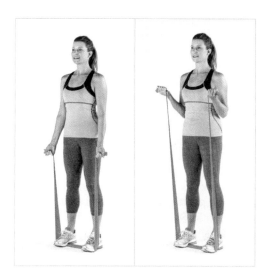

⑪ Arm extensions

Muscles worked: Triceps

Reps: 8–12 with each arm for strength,
  6–10 with each arm for power
Sets: 1–3
Tempo: 3–1–3 for strength,
  1–1–3 for power
Rest: 30–90 seconds between sets

Starting position: Stand tall and hold one end of the band in your right hand. Raise your right arm overhead and bend your elbow, lowering your right hand behind your head with the band hanging behind your back. Bend your left arm behind your back so you can grasp the hanging part of the band with your left hand.

Movement: Extend your right arm, raising your right hand overhead. Keep your upper arm stationary and your arm close to your head. Slowly lower to the starting position. This is one rep. Finish all reps, then repeat with your left arm. This completes one set.

Tips and techniques:
• Don't move from your shoulder. The movement is at your elbow.

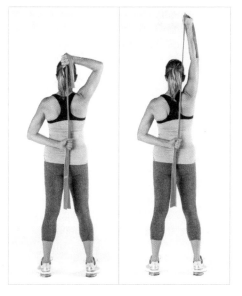

• Keep your shoulders down and back, away from your ears.
• Keep your wrists straight, in line with your arms.

Make it easier: Place your hands farther apart on the band for less resistance, or use a lighter resistance band.

Make it harder: Place your hands closer together on the band for more resistance, or use a heavier resistance band. ◗

QUICK RESISTANCE BAND WORKOUT

On days when you feel that you just don't have time for a full workout, do this abbreviated routine. Some exercise is better than none!

• **Chest press** (page 29)
• **Seated row with rotation** (page 30)
• **Leg press** (page 30)
• **Ab crunch with band** (page 31)

Medicine Ball Workout

You should have some strength training under your belt before trying this workout. While you can modify the moves, it is still an advanced routine that combines both strength and power in many of the moves. This makes it a time-efficient workout, but also a more intense one. You may notice that your heart rate goes up more than during other strength workouts.

For a demonstration of the plank pass (page 37), go to the video at www.health.harvard.edu/plank-pass.

① Squat and overhead toss

Muscles worked: Quadriceps, hamstrings, gluteus, pectoralis, deltoids, biceps, erector spinae

Reps: 6–10
Sets: 1–3
Tempo: 3–1–1
Rest: 30–90 seconds between sets

Starting position: Stand tall with your feet about shoulder-width apart, toes pointed out slightly. Hold a medicine ball with both hands at chest height, arms bent.

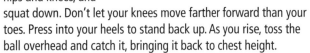

Movement: Bend your hips and knees, and squat down. Don't let your knees move farther forward than your toes. Press into your heels to stand back up. As you rise, toss the ball overhead and catch it, bringing it back to chest height.

Tips and techniques:
• Keep your chest lifted to avoid leaning too far forward.

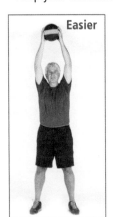
Easier

• Start with a small toss. Gradually throw the ball higher as you become more comfortable with the exercise.

◄ **Make it easier:** Do the move without the toss. Instead, simply extend your arms, raising the ball overhead. Use a lighter medicine ball.

Make it harder: Squat lower and extend your arms, touching the ball to the floor, and toss the ball higher. Use a heavier medicine ball.

② Crunch

Muscles worked: Rectus abdominis, transverse abdominis, psoas major, pectoralis, deltoids, triceps

Reps: 8–12
Sets: 1–3
Tempo: 3–1–3
Rest: 30–90 seconds between sets

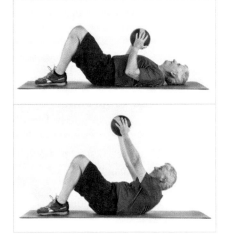

Starting position: Lie faceup on the floor with your legs bent and your feet flat on the floor. Hold a medicine ball close to your chest, elbows pointing out to the sides.

Movement: Contract your abdominal muscles and curl your head, shoulders, and upper back off the floor. Simultaneously, extend your arms, thrusting the ball out in front of you. Hold, and then lower.

Tips and techniques:
• Look straight ahead, not up at the ceiling or down at your belly, as you crunch.
• Keep your mid-back on the mat.
• Don't hold your breath.

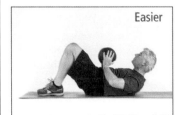
Easier

◄ **Make it easier:** Hold the ball by your chest for the entire move. Don't extend your arms. Use a lighter medicine ball.

Make it harder: Hold in the "up" position for three to five seconds. Use a heavier medicine ball.

③ Overhead floor slam

Muscles worked: Deltoids, latissimus dorsi, rectus abdominis, quadriceps, hamstrings, gluteus, triceps

Reps: 6–10
Sets: 1–3
Tempo: 1–1
Rest: 30–90 seconds between sets

Starting position: Stand tall with your feet about hip-width apart, toes pointing straight ahead. Hold a medicine ball with both hands at chest height, arms bent.

Movement: Extend your arms and bring the ball overhead. In a smooth motion, bring the ball down in front of you as you bend your hips and knees and throw the ball to the floor as hard as possible. Keep your arms straight. Squat down to pick up the ball and return to the starting position.

Tips and techniques:
• Keep your chest lifted.
• Don't bend at your waist.
• Keep your knees no farther forward than your toes.

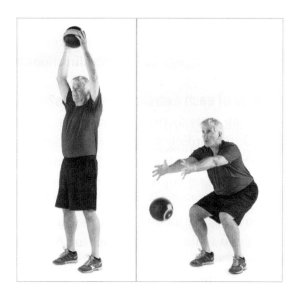

Make it easier: Instead of slamming the ball to the floor, simply let it drop.

Make it harder: Use a heavier medicine ball.

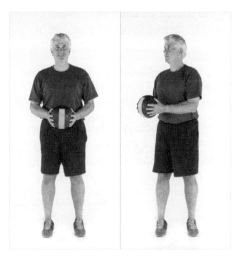

④ Twists

Muscles worked: Obliques

Reps: 8–12
Sets: 1–3
Tempo: 3–1–3
Rest: 30–90 seconds between sets

Starting position: Stand tall with your feet about hip-width apart, toes pointing straight ahead. Hold a medicine ball with both hands at waist height, arms bent.

Movement: Slowly rotate to the right as far as is comfortable, turning your head to follow. Return to the center. Rotate to the left. This is one rep.

Tips and techniques:
• Keep your feet flat on the floor.
• Don't rotate your head farther than your arms.
• Keep your abs tight.

Harder

   Make it easier: Use a lighter medicine ball. Don't rotate as far.

◀ **Make it harder:** Extend your arms out in front of you and twist. Use a heavier medicine ball.

⑤ One-leg dead lift

Muscles worked: Gluteus, hamstrings

Reps: 8–12 with each leg
Sets: 1–3
Tempo: 3–1–3
Rest: 30–90 seconds between sets

Starting position: Stand tall with your feet together, toes pointing straight ahead. Hold a medicine ball with both hands, arms extended down in front of you.

Movement: Shift your weight to your left foot. Slowly raise your right leg behind you as your upper body hinges forward at the hips, lowering the ball toward the floor. Hold. Press into your supporting leg to return to the starting position. Finish all reps, then repeat on the other side. This completes one set.

Tips and techniques:
- Keep your hips level.
- Don't lock the knee of your standing leg.
- Lower only until your torso and back leg are parallel to the floor.

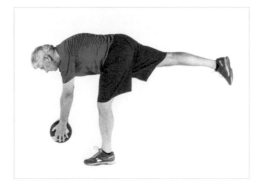

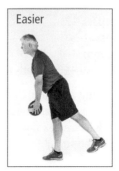

Easier

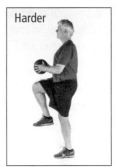

Harder

▶ **Make it easier:** Hinge forward only about 45 degrees. Use a lighter medicine ball.

▶ **Make it harder:** As you stand back up, bring your back leg forward and up into a knee lift before returning to the starting position. Use a heavier medicine ball.

⑥ Reverse crunch

Muscles worked: Rectus abdominis, transverse abdominis, psoas major, adductors

Reps: 8–12
Sets: 1–3
Tempo: 1–1–2
Rest: 30–90 seconds between sets

Starting position: Lie faceup on the floor with your legs bent and your feet off the floor. Place a medicine ball between your knees, making sure that it is secure.

Movement: Squeeze the ball with your thighs. Contract your abdominal muscles and lift your buttocks and hips off the floor, bringing your knees toward you. Hold, and then slowly lower. If the ball feels insecure, you can place one hand on it to prevent it from falling on you.

Tips and techniques:
- Keep the movement slow and controlled.

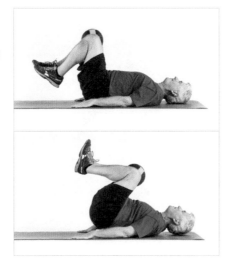

- Don't hold your breath.

Make it easier: Use a lighter medicine ball or none at all.

Make it harder: Hold in the "up" position for three to five seconds. Use a heavier medicine ball.

QUICK MEDICINE BALL WORKOUT

On days when you feel that you just don't have time for a full workout, do this abbreviated routine. Some exercise is better than none!

- **Squat and overhead toss** (page 34)
- **Overhead floor slam** (page 35)
- **Plank pass** (page 37)
- **Lunge and lift** (page 37)

(7) Plank pass

Muscles worked: *Deltoids, erector spinae, rectus abdominis, gluteus, transverse abdominis*

Reps: 8–12
Sets: 1–3
Tempo: 1–1
Rest: 30–90 seconds between sets

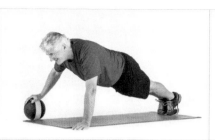
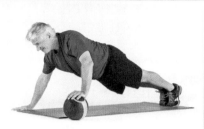

Starting position: Begin on the floor on all fours with your hands about shoulder-width apart and the medicine ball by your right hand. Lift your knees off the floor and straighten your legs behind you.

Movement: Shift your weight to your left hand so you can place your right hand on the ball. Roll the ball to the left, placing your right hand down and lifting your left hand to stop the ball. Then, roll it to the right. This is one rep.

Tips and techniques:
• Keep your body in line from your head to your heels.
• Keep your abs tight to prevent your back from arching too much.
• Don't drop your head.

Easier
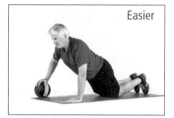

Harder
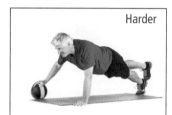

◄ **Make it easier:** Do the move with your knees on the floor. When you've mastered that, lift up into the full plank each time you catch the ball—one hand on the ball and one on the floor. Then, lower your knees to the floor to roll and catch the ball before lifting up into the full plank again. Try holding the full plank a little longer over time until you feel strong enough to do the unmodified move.

◄ **Make it harder:** Place one foot on top of the other to do the move in a one-leg plank position.

(8) Lunge and lift

Muscles worked: *Gluteus, quadriceps, hamstrings, triceps*

Reps: 8–12
Sets: 1–3
Tempo: 4–1
Rest: 30–90 seconds between sets

Starting position: Stand up straight with your feet together and hold a medicine ball with both hands, with your hands down in front of you.

Movement: Step back onto the ball of your right foot, as you raise the ball over your head. Bend your knees, and lower into a lunge, while simultaneously bending your elbows and lowering the ball behind your head. Your left knee should align with your left ankle, and your right knee should point toward the floor. Push off your back foot to stand up, straightening your arms and raising the ball overhead, and return to the starting position. Repeat on the opposite side, stepping back with your left foot to do the lunge. This is one rep.

Tips and techniques:
• Keep your spine neutral when lowering into the lunge.
• Don't lean forward.

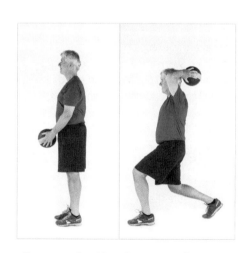

• Keep your shoulders down, away from your ears.

Make it easier: Use a lighter medicine ball. Another option is to do stationary lunges instead of stepping back and forth: Stand with one foot in front of the other and lower into the lunge. Finish all reps, then switch legs and repeat for one set.

Make it harder: Step forward into the lunge instead of backward, and as you stand back up do a knee lift. Use a heavier medicine ball. ▼

Kettlebell Workout

Get ready for a trio of benefits from the Kettlebell Workout. Like the Medicine Ball Workout (page 34), this routine contains moves that build both strength and power. But you'll also get a heart-pumping cardio workout because of the vigorous actions of many of the exercises. It is important that you practice these moves without a kettlebell at first, so that you learn good tech-nique to avoid injury. You should also start by doing the moves at a slower tempo and gradually progress to the paces noted in the exercise instructions.

For further advice on how to perform kettlebell exercises properly, getting maximum benefits while minimizing your risk of injury, go to the video at www.health.harvard.edu/kettlebell.

(1) Basic swing

Muscles worked: Deltoids, erector spinae, gluteus, quadriceps, hamstrings

Reps: 8–12
Sets: 1–3
Tempo: 1–1
Rest: 30–90 seconds between sets

Starting position: Stand tall with your feet about shoulder-width apart. Hold a kettlebell with both hands, arms extended down in front of you so the kettlebell hangs between your legs.

Movement: Hinge forward at your hips, shift your weight onto your heels, and sit back, swinging the kettlebell back between your legs. Then press into your heels and stand up as you swing the kettlebell forward to chest height.

Tips and techniques:
• Keep your abs tight.
• Don't round your back or bend at the waist.
• Don't push your hips out in front of your body or lean back as you stand up.

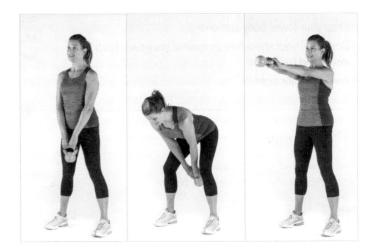

Make it easier: Use a lighter kettlebell.

▶ **Make it harder:** Hold the kettlebell in one hand and pass it to the other as you swing it.

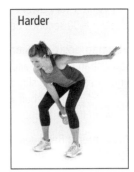

Harder

② Halo

Muscles worked: Rectus abdominis, obliques, transverse abdominis, deltoids

Reps: 8–12
Sets: 1–3
Tempo: 3
Rest: 30–90 seconds between sets

Starting position: Stand with your feet about shoulder-width apart. Hold a kettlebell with both hands so it is over and behind your head.

Movement: Circle the kettlebell clockwise over your head for half of the repetitions. Then circle counterclockwise for the remaining repetitions. This completes one set.

Tips and techniques:

• Keep your lower body stationary.
• Don't pull your shoulders up toward your ears; keep them down and back.
• Keep your abs tight.

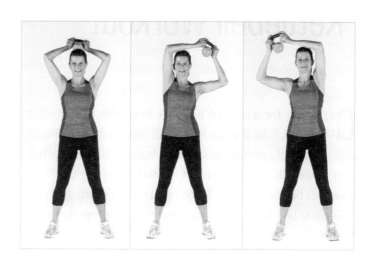

Make it easier: Make smaller circles, or use a lighter kettlebell.

Make it harder: Make larger circles, or use a heavier kettlebell.

③ High pull

Muscles worked: Gluteus, quadriceps, hamstrings, erector spinae, deltoids, biceps

Reps: 8–12
Sets: 1–3
Tempo: 3–1–3–1 for strength,
  1–1–1–1 for power
Rest: 30–90 seconds between sets

Starting position: Stand with your feet more than shoulder-width apart and your toes pointing slightly out to the sides. Hold a kettlebell with both hands down in front of you.

Movement: Bend your knees and hips, lowering into a squat. Hold. As you stand up, bend your elbows out to the sides and pull the kettlebell up to about chest height. Hold again. This is one rep.

Tips and techniques:

• Don't let your knees roll in as you squat.

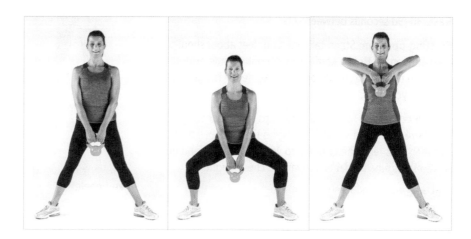

• Keep your abs tight.
• Your knees should move no farther forward than your toes as you squat.

  Make it easier: Do the pull without squatting.

▶ **Make it harder:** Hold the kettlebell in one hand only and do the pulls with one arm at a time.

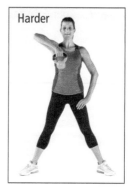

Harder

④ Lunge press

Muscles worked: Deltoids, erector spinae, triceps, rectus abdominis, obliques, gluteus, quadriceps, hamstrings

Reps: 8–12
Sets: 1–3
Tempo: 3–1–3 for strength, 2-1–1 for power
Rest: 30–90 seconds between sets

Starting position: Stand with your feet together and hold a kettlebell with both hands by your chest.

Movement: Step back onto the ball of your left foot, bend your knees, and lower into a lunge. At the same time, extend your arms and press the kettlebell overhead. Your right knee should align over your right ankle, and your left knee should point toward the floor. Hold. Push off your back foot to stand up and return to the starting position. Repeat, stepping back with your right foot to do the lunge on the opposite side. This is one rep.

Tips and techniques:
• Keep your spine neutral when lowering into the lunge.
• Don't lean forward or back.

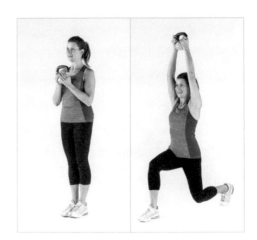

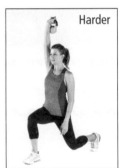

Harder

• As you bend your knees, lower the back knee directly down toward the floor, with the thigh perpendicular to the floor.

   Make it easier: Do the lunge without pressing the kettlebell overhead.

▶ **Make it harder:** Hold the kettlebell in one hand to do the presses with one arm at a time.

⑤ Windmill

Muscles worked: Obliques

Reps: 8–12 on each side
Sets: 1–3
Tempo: 3–1–3 for strength, 3–1–1 for power
Rest: 30–90 seconds between sets

Starting position: Stand tall with your feet more than shoulder-width apart. Hold a kettlebell in your left hand with your left arm extended overhead, and your right arm down at your side.

Movement: Slowly bend to your right side as far as is comfortable. Let your right hand slide down your right leg as you lower. Look up at your left hand. Hold. Slowly return to the starting position. Finish all reps, then repeat on the opposite side. This completes one set.

Tips and techniques:
• Don't let your body roll forward as you bend.
• Keep your abs tight.
• Don't twist your neck too far.

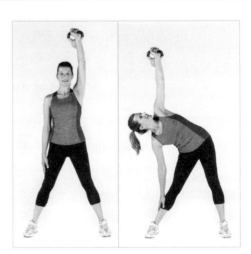

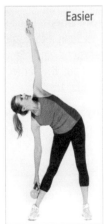

Easier

▶ **Make it easier:** Hold the kettlebell in your other hand, down at your side, instead of over your head.

   Make it harder: Hold a kettlebell in each hand.

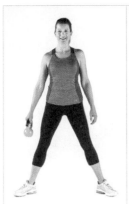 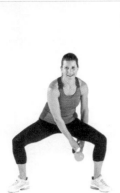 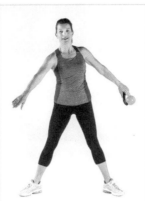 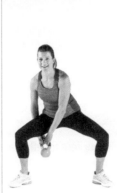 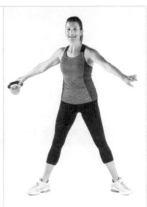

⑥ Figure eight

Muscles worked: Deltoids, erector spinae, rectus abdominis, obliques

Reps: 8–12 in each direction
Sets: 1–3
Tempo: 1–1–1–1
Rest: 30–90 seconds between sets

Starting position: Stand tall with your feet more than shoulder-width apart. Hold a kettlebell in your right hand with your right arm at your side.

Movement: Bend your knees and bring the kettlebell around the front of your right leg and pass it between your legs to your left hand. Straighten up as you bring the

kettlebell around in front to your left leg, and squat again to pass it between your legs back to your right hand. This is one rep. Finish all reps, then repeat going in the opposite direction. This completes one set.

Tips and techniques:
• Keep your abs tight.
• Be careful that you don't hit your legs as you pass the kettlebell between them.
• Maintain control.

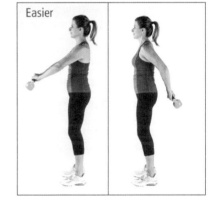

Easier

▶ **Make it easier:** Circle the kettlebell around your waist. Or, use a lighter kettlebell.

Make it harder: Use a heavier kettlebell, or squat lower.

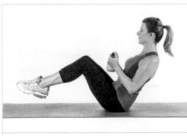

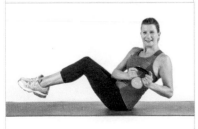

⑦ Seated twist

Muscles worked: Rectus abdominis, obliques, transverse abdominis, erector spinae

Reps: 8–12
Sets: 1–3
Tempo: 2–2–2–2 for strength,
1–1–1–1 for power
Rest: 30–90 seconds between sets

Starting position: Sit on the floor with your knees bent and feet on the floor. Hold a kettlebell with both hand in front of your chest. Shift your weight onto your tailbone and raise your feet off the floor.

Movement: Slowly twist to the left. Hold. Return to the center, and then twist to the right. This is one rep.

Tips and techniques:
• Keep your chest lifted.
• Don't lean back too far.
• Don't hold your breath.

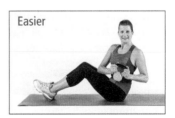

Easier

▶ **Make it easier:** Keep your heels on the floor. Use a lighter kettlebell.

Make it harder: Raise your feet higher off the floor. Use a heavier kettlebell.

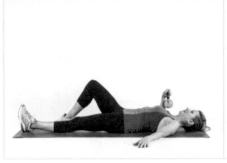 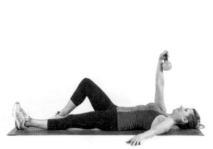 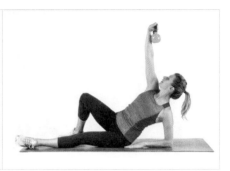

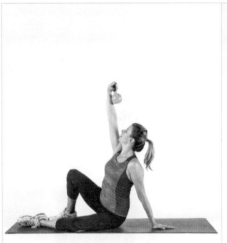 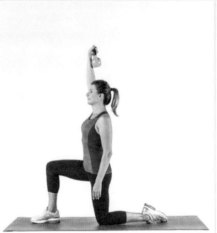 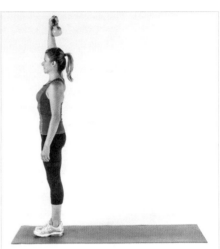

⑧ Get up

Muscles worked: Pectoralis, triceps, deltoids, erector spinae, rectus abdominis, gluteus, quadriceps, hamstrings

Reps: 4–6 on each side
Sets: 1–3 on each side
Tempo: 1–1–1–1–1
Rest: 30–90 seconds between sets

Starting position: Lie faceup on the floor with your right leg bent, foot flat on the floor, and your left leg extended. Hold a kettlebell in your right hand with your right arm bent, elbow pointing out to the side and upper arm resting on the floor.

Movement: Extend your right arm, pressing the kettlebell straight up to the ceiling. Curl your head and torso off the floor, rising up onto your left elbow and forearm. Shift onto your left hand, sitting up further. Shift your weight onto your right foot and slide your left leg

back and under your torso, rising up onto your left knee. Press into your right foot to stand up, bringing your feet together. Hold, and then slowly reverse the moves, returning to the starting position. Complete all reps on one side, then repeat with the opposite arm and leg.

Tips and techniques:
• Exhale as you exert effort.
• Keep your abs tight.
• Maintain control.

Make it easier: Rise only to the seated position.

Make it harder: Try using a heavier kettlebell. ◥

QUICK KETTLEBELL WORKOUT

On days when you feel that you just don't have time for a full workout, do this abbreviated routine. Some exercise is better than none!

• **Basic swing** (page 38)
• **High pull** (page 39)
• **Seated twist** (page 41)
• **Get up** (page 42)

Bonus power moves: Plyometrics

Adding a few of these moves to any strength workout that you do will boost your power by training your fast-twitch muscle fibers (see "Slow-twitch and fast-twitch fibers," page 7), the nerves that activate them, and your reflexes. If you have never done plyometrics or jump training, start with the beginner moves. Even if you have some experience with this type of exercise, that's still a good place to start, and then you can progress to the other levels more quickly.

Perform plyometrics at the beginning of your training session—but *after* you are warmed up. Do three sets of five reps for each move, allowing at least a minute of rest in between sets. If this is too much for you, you can do fewer reps or sets. Over time, gradually work up to 15 reps per set. Aim to do plyometrics one to three times a week, allowing 48 to 72 hours in between sessions for adequate recovery. When you are ready for a new challenge, try the next level of jumps, starting with three sets of five reps and progressing from there.

Here are some tips to maximize your efforts while minimizing your risk for injury:

- Choose a surface with some give. A thick, firm mat (not the yoga kind); well-padded, carpeted wood floor; or grass or dirt, outside, are good choices that absorb some of the impact. Do not jump on tile, concrete, or asphalt surfaces.
- Jump slowly in the beginning. The faster you jump, the more intense the workout.
- Aim for just a few inches off the floor to start. The higher you jump, the greater your impact on landing.
- Bend your legs when you land. Don't lock your knees.
- Land softly on your midfoot, not your heels or balls of your feet.
- Drop your hips as you land to absorb some of the impact.
- Engage your core muscles to protect your spine.
- Lean slightly forward, with your head up and your torso rigid (chest over knees, nose over toes) as you land.
- If you have had any joint issues, especially in your knees, back, or hips, check with your doctor before doing any plyometric training.

BEGINNER: Knee hops

Muscles worked: Gluteus, quadriceps, hamstrings, gastrocnemius

Reps: 5–15 with each leg
Sets: 1–3
Rest: 1 to 3 minutes between sets

Starting position: Stand tall with your feet together.

Movement: Raise your left knee up to about hip height, hopping a little bit off the floor with your right foot as you lift. Immediately repeat with your opposite leg. Continue alternating legs. Let your arms swing naturally.

Tips and techniques:
- Don't hunch or round your shoulders forward.
- Keep your abs tight.

Make it easier: Don't lift your knee as high. Don't hop as high, or keep your toes on the floor as you raise your heel.

Make it harder: Lift your knee higher. Hop higher.

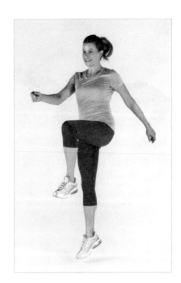

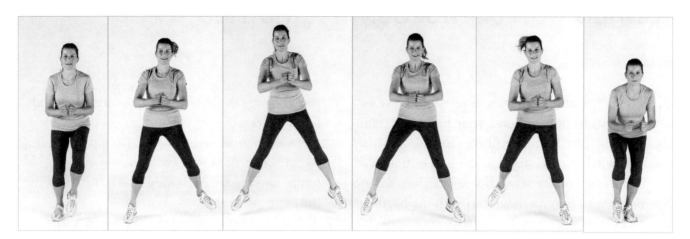

BEGINNER: Side hops

Muscles worked: *Gluteus, abductors, adductors, quadriceps, hamstrings, gastrocnemius*

Reps: 5–15 to each side
Sets: 1   3
Rest: 1 to 3 minutes between sets

Starting position: Stand tall with your feet together.

Movement: Shift your weight onto your right foot and leap to your left, landing with your left foot followed by your right one. Repeat, hopping to your right. You can hold your arms in front of you or let them swing naturally.

Tips and techniques:
- Don't hunch or round your shoulders forward.
- Keep your abs tight.

Make it easier: Hop a shorter distance to the side and stay lower to the floor.

Make it harder: Make your hops bigger and higher.

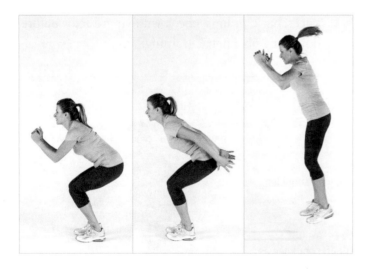

INTERMEDIATE: Forward and backward hops

Muscles worked: *Gluteus, quadriceps, hamstrings, gastrocnemius*

Reps: 5–15
Sets: 1–3
Rest: 1 to 3 minutes between sets

Starting position: Stand tall with your feet together.

Movement: Bend your knees and jump forward one to two feet. Then jump back to the starting position. Let your arms swing naturally.

Tips and techniques:
- Don't hunch or round your shoulders forward.
- Keep your abs tight.

Make it easier: Hop a shorter distance and stay lower to the floor.

Make it harder: Make your hops longer and higher.

INTERMEDIATE: Jumping jacks

Muscles worked: Deltoids, gluteus, quadriceps, hamstrings, gastrocnemius

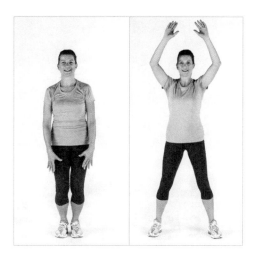

Reps: 5–15
Sets: 1–3
Rest: 1 to 3 minutes between sets

Starting position: Stand tall with your feet together, arms at your sides.

Movement: Jump and spread your feet apart, more than shoulder-width, as you raise your arms out to the sides and over your head. Jump and bring your feet back together, bringing your arms down to your sides. This is one rep.

Tips and techniques:
• Don't hunch or round your shoulders forward.
• Keep your abs tight.

Make it easier: Don't move your feet as far apart, and stay lower to the floor.

Make it harder: Make your jumps higher and faster.

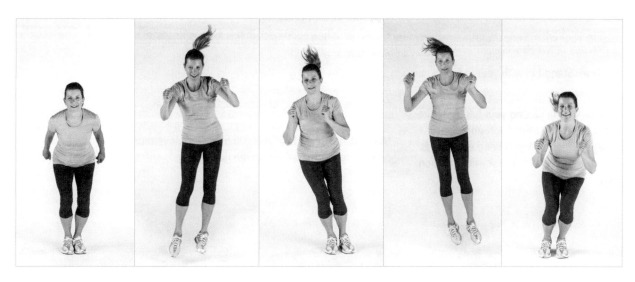

ADVANCED: Lateral jumps

Muscles worked: Gluteus, abductors, quadriceps, hamstrings, gastrocnemius

Reps: 5–15
Sets: 1–3
Rest: 1 to 3 minutes between sets

Starting position: Stand tall with your feet together, arms at your sides.

Movement: Bend your knees and jump to your left with both feet. Then jump back to the starting position. This is one rep.

Tips and techniques:
• Don't hunch or round your shoulders forward.
• Keep your abs tight.

Make it easier: Jump a shorter distance and stay lower to the floor.

Make it harder: Make your jumps longer, higher, or faster.

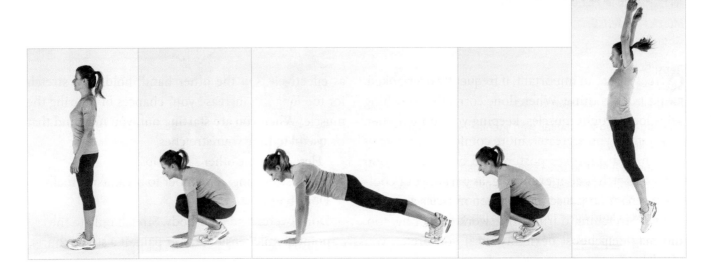

ADVANCED: Burpees

Muscles worked: Deltoids, pectoralis, rectus abdominis, transverse abdominis, erector spinae, gluteus, quadriceps, hamstrings, gastrocnemius

Reps: 5–15
Sets: 1–3
Rest: 1 to 3 minutes between sets

Starting position: Stand tall with your feet together, arms at your sides.

Movement: Squat down placing your hands on the floor. Jump your legs back behind you into plank position. Jump your feet back in toward your hands. Jump up into the air, landing in the starting position. This is one rep.

Tips and techniques:
• Keep your head and neck in line with your spine.
• Keep your abs tight.

Make it easier: Walk your feet in and out of the plank position instead of jumping. Don't jump as high.

Make it harder: Make your jump higher. Move more quickly from one position to the next. ▼

Stretching exercises

Stretching is an important, if frequently overlooked, part of a routine. When done correctly, stretching helps loosen tight muscles, keeping you more limber. It also gives you a greater, more comfortable range of motion and improves posture and balance. A good time to stretch is after exercising, as part of your cool-down session, because that is when muscles are most pliable. Stretching during your workout is fine, too, and may help boost flexibility, so if you prefer, you can do a stretch or two after each exercise once your muscles are warmed up.

To perform the stretches: Be sure to hold each stretch for 10 to 30 seconds and repeat it three or four times. If you hold the position for less time or do fewer repetitions, you won't lengthen the muscle fibers as effectively. On the other hand, holding a stretch for too long can increase your chances of injuring the muscle. When you are starting out, you may find that it's useful to time your stretches.

Here are some other safety tips:
• While stretching, remember to breathe normally.
• Don't bounce.
• Don't overextend your body. Stretch only to the point of mild tension, never pain. If a stretch hurts, stop immediately.

If you have had a joint replaced or repaired, ask your surgeon whether you need to avoid certain stretches, such as the torso rotation. If you have osteoporosis, consult your doctor before doing floor stretches or stretches that bend the spine.

Chest opener

Where you'll feel it: Chest and shoulders

Reps: 2–6
Hold: 10–30 seconds

Starting position: Stand with your feet together and your arms at your sides.

Movement: Clasp your hands together behind you. Gently raise your hands as high as is comfortable, pulling your shoulders back and opening up your chest. Hold. Return to the starting position.

Tips and techniques:
• If you have difficulty clasping your hands, hold on to a towel or strap with both hands.
• Keep your shoulders down and back.
• Don't lean forward or excessively arch your back.

Triceps stretch

Where you'll feel it: Back of upper arm

Reps: 2–6
Hold: 10–30 seconds

Starting position: Stand with your feet comfortably apart and your arms at your sides.

Movement: Raise your right arm overhead and bend your elbow so your right hand is behind your head. Place your left hand on your right elbow and gently pull it toward the left. Hold. Slowly return to the starting position. Repeat with your left arm behind your head. This is one rep.

Tips and techniques:
• Keep your chest lifted and your eyes straight ahead.
• Keep your back straight and your shoulders down and back.
• Don't lean to the side.

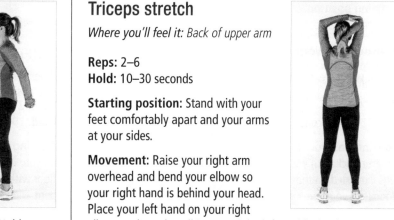

Calf stretch

Where you'll feel it: Back of lower leg, ankle, top of thigh

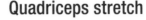

Reps: 2–6
Hold: 10–30 seconds

Starting position: Stand up straight with your feet together and your hands on your hips or down at your sides.

Movement: Step with your left foot 12 to 24 inches behind you and bend your right knee. Keeping both feet flat, press your left heel against the floor as you lean forward from the ankle. Hold. Return to the starting position, then repeat with your right leg back. This is one rep.

Tips and techniques:
• Keep your toes pointing forward.
• Your hips and shoulders should remain squared, facing forward.
• If you don't feel a stretch, place your foot farther back.

Quadriceps stretch

Where you'll feel it: Front of thigh

Reps: 2–6
Hold: 10–30 seconds

Starting position: Stand with your feet together. Place your right hand on the back of a chair for balance if needed.

Movement: Bend your left knee and bring your heel toward your left buttock. Grasp your left foot with your left hand. Hold. Slowly return to the starting position. Repeat on the other side. This is one rep.

Tips and techniques:
• Don't grasp your toes.
• If you have trouble reaching your foot, loop a strap or belt around your ankle and gently pull the strap toward your buttocks.
• Don't arch your back.
• Make sure your bent knee is pointing straight down toward the floor.
• Tuck your tailbone under to feel a deeper stretch.

Knees to chest

Where you'll feel it: Lower and middle back, hips

Reps: 2–6
Hold: 10–30 seconds

Starting position: Lie on your back with your legs extended on the floor. Rest your arms at your sides.

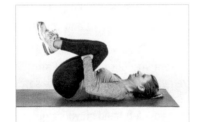

Movement: Bend both knees and grasp them from behind with your hands, pulling them in toward your chest. Hold. Return to the starting position.

Tips and techniques:
• Bring your chin to your chest for a greater stretch.
• When holding the stretch, remain as still as possible.

Lying pretzel

Where you'll feel it: Buttocks, hip, and outer thigh

Reps: 2–6
Hold: 10–30 seconds

Starting position: Lie on your back on the floor with your knees bent and your feet flat.

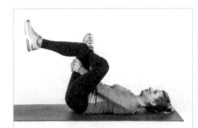

Movement: Place your left ankle across your right thigh just above the knee. Grasp your right leg behind the thigh and gently pull it in toward your chest until you feel mild tension in your left hip and buttock. Hold. Slowly return to the starting position. Repeat with your right foot across your left thigh. This is one rep.

Tips and techniques:
• Keep your head on the floor.
• Keep your hips squared; don't let them roll to one side.
• For a deeper stretch, use your hand to press your bent leg away from you.

Torso rotation*

Where you'll feel it: Back, chest, and outer thigh

Reps: 2–6
Hold: 10–30 seconds

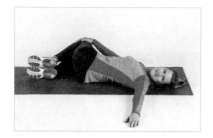

Starting position:
Lie on your back with your knees bent and feet together, flat on the floor. Extend your arms out comfortably to each side at shoulder level.

Movement: Tighten your abdominal muscles and slowly lower your knees to the right side, keeping them together and resting them on the floor. Keep your shoulders relaxed and pressed against the floor as you turn your head in the opposite direction, looking toward your left hand. You can place your right hand on your left thigh to deepen the stretch. Hold. Return to the starting position. Repeat in the opposite direction. This is one rep.

Tips and techniques:

- When holding the stretch, remain as still as possible, without bouncing.
- If it's too difficult to rest your knees on the floor, place a folded blanket on the floor and rest them on it.
- If necessary, put a rolled towel between your knees to make this stretch easier.

* If you have had a hip replacement, talk to your doctor before trying this stretch. It may be best for you to avoid it.

Hamstring stretch

Where you'll feel it: Back of thigh

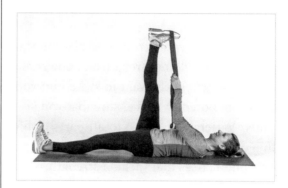

Reps: 2–6
Hold: 10–30 seconds

Starting position: Lie on your back on the floor with your legs extended. Loop a strap or belt around your right foot and grasp the ends.

Movement: Raise your right leg off the floor as high as possible. Then gently pull on the strap to bring your right leg in toward your chest as far as you comfortably can. Hold. Slowly return to the starting position. Repeat with your left leg. This is one rep.

Tips and techniques:

- Keep your legs straight, but don't lock your knees.
- If you don't have a strap or you prefer not to use one, you can grasp the back of your thigh with both hands.
- If you feel any strain or are unable to maintain good form, you can bend the opposite leg and place that foot flat on the floor. ♦

More ways to get strong

The workouts in this report are a good place to start when it comes to building strength and power. But at some point, you will likely want to switch up your routine to prevent boredom and ensure that you keep seeing results. Variety adds spice to all parts of life, and working out is no different. Here are some popular workouts and classes that include strength training, power training, or both. In some cases they also include cardio or flexibility benefits.

Barre classes. Exercises are performed at a ballet barre and focus on strengthening individual muscle groups while improving flexibility, posture, and balance. No power training here.

BodyPump/body sculpting classes. Group strength training workouts are set to music to make lifting weights more fun. The focus tends to be on using light weights for many repetitions to build endurance. Some strength benefits may be possible depending upon your fitness level.

Boot camps. Military-inspired workouts, done outdoors or indoors, get your heart pumping for cardio benefits and work your muscles for both strength and power gains.

CrossFit. A regimen of high-intensity interval training provides cardio, strength, and power training. Because of its vigorous nature (flipping tires and hefting very heavy weights), proceed with caution if you decide to try it.

Heavy ropes. More and more gyms are offering giant-sized ropes, attached to an anchor point, as a novel way to build upper-body strength and power. Depending upon the moves you do, you could also get a bit of a cardio workout.

Kickboxing/boxing. Punching and kicking during this high-energy cardio workout helps to build

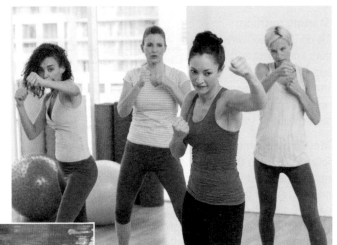

© Wavebreakmedia | Thinkstock

There are many options for strength and power training. Water workouts give you both strength and cardio benefits. Boxing and kickboxing help develop power.

power. It can improve speed and agility, which are components of power, but it doesn't offer much in the way of strength training.

Martial arts. High-energy styles of martial arts with jumps, kicks, and blocks can provide cardio, strength, and power benefits. Most classes also include stretching for a well-rounded workout.

Ninja Warrior/Tough Mudder workouts. As these competitive obstacle-course-style races have gained popularity, workouts to train for them have popped up. These hard-core workouts generally hit all the fitness components—cardio, strength, power, flexibility—with an emphasis on strength.

Pilates. Equipment includes weighted hand balls, resistance bands or straps, and machines with pulleys, cables, and straps for resistance. But even Pilates classes done on a mat with no equipment can help you get stronger. No cardio or power benefits, however.

Step aerobics. Hopping and stepping up and down during this cardio workout can provide some lower-body strength gains. And the more hopping and jumping over the step you do, the more power training you'll get.

TRX. This unique body-weight workout uses straps that are anchored overhead to suspend you as you do the exercises. It's a strength workout that really works your core. Some moves may also provide power benefits.

Water workouts. Water provides resistance, so you get both cardio and strength benefits when you hop in the pool. And if you're doing moves like running and jumping, you may also get some power benefits.

Yoga. Holding poses helps to build strength and muscle endurance, while flowing stretches increase flexibility. Some vigorous styles of yoga, such as Ashtanga, may provide some cardio benefits. ◗

Resources

Organizations

American Academy of Physical Medicine and Rehabilitation
9700 W. Bryn Mawr Ave., Suite 200
Rosemont, IL 60018
847-737-6000
www.aapmr.org

This national organization is for doctors who specialize in physical medicine and rehabilitation for musculoskeletal and neurological problems. AAPMR offers referrals to these doctors and information on a variety of conditions such as low back and neck pain, spinal cord and brain injuries, osteoporosis, and arthritis.

American College of Sports Medicine
401 W. Michigan St.
Indianapolis, IN 46206
317-637-9200
www.acsm.org

This nonprofit organization is devoted to expanding scientific knowledge about exercise and developing programs for health and exercise professionals. ACSM offers several types of certification in sports medicine, health, and fitness for health and exercise professionals as well as information on strength and power training and other forms of exercise for the general public.

American Council on Exercise
4851 Paramount Drive
San Diego, CA 92123
888-825-3636 (toll-free)
www.acefitness.org

This nonprofit organization promotes fitness and a healthy lifestyle. ACE certifies fitness professionals and also offers educational materials and consumer information on finding and evaluating personal trainers and health coaches.

American Physical Therapy Association
1111 N. Fairfax St.
Alexandria, VA 22314
800-999-2782 (toll-free)
www.apta.org

This national professional organization fosters advances in education, research, and the practice of physical therapy. APTA's website has a search engine to help locate board-certified clinical specialists who have additional training in specific areas of physical therapy.

Special Health Reports

The following Special Health Reports from Harvard Medical School will give you more exercises to expand your program in different ways. Order online at www.health.harvard.edu or call 877-649-9457 (toll-free).

Core Exercises: 5 workouts to tighten your abs, strengthen your back, and improve your balance
Lauren E. Elson, Medical Editor, with Michele Stanten, Fitness Consultant
(Harvard Medical School, 2016)

Stretching: 35 stretches to improve flexibility and reduce pain
Lauren E. Elson, Medical Editor, with Josie Gardiner, Personal Trainer
(Harvard Medical School, 2014)

Walking for Health: Why this simple form of exercise could be your best health insurance
Lauren E. Elson, Medical Editor, with Michele Stanten, Fitness Consultant
(Harvard Medical School, 2015)

Workout Workbook: 9 complete workouts to help you get fit and healthy
Lauren E. Elson, Medical Editor, with Michele Stanten, Fitness Consultant
(Harvard Medical School, 2016)

Glossary

aerobic activity: An activity or exercise that increases heart rate and breathing through repetitive use of large muscles, such as walking, running, or biking. Also known as endurance exercise, aerobic activity conditions the heart, lungs, circulatory system, and muscles.

concentric action: When muscles exert force and move joints by shortening.

eccentric action: When muscles exert force and move joints by lengthening.

fast-twitch fiber: One of two main types of skeletal muscle fibers. Fast-twitch fibers are recruited most heavily when bursts of power are needed, as in sprinting.

isometric (static) action: When muscles generate force, but neither contract nor extend enough to move a joint (such as when someone pushes against an immovable object).

motor neuron: A nerve cell that directs activity in a specific group of muscle fibers.

motor unit: The pairing of a nerve cell and the group of muscle fibers it commands.

muscle fibers: Cells that are bundled together to make up muscle tissue. Also known as muscle cells.

myofibrils: Long interlocking strands that make up muscle fibers.

myofilaments: The fundamental muscle proteins that form myofibrils. Myofilaments slide over one another, bunching up and generating force, when a muscle contracts.

power: Force times speed of movement. It reflects how quickly a force is exerted.

power training: An emerging field of physical medicine aimed at boosting the ability to exert strength quickly, especially in relation to practical, day-to-day tasks.

repetitions (reps): Number of times an exercise calls for a muscle to be worked and released (usually eight to 12).

set: A given number of repetitions of an exercise.

skeletal muscles: Muscles attached to bones throughout the body that allow voluntary movement to occur.

slow-twitch fiber: One of two main types of skeletal muscle fibers. Slow-twitch fibers are recruited most heavily for endurance (aerobic) exercises.

strength: The ability to exert force.

strength training: Popular term for exercises that harness resistance supplied by body weight, free weights such as dumbbells, or specialized machines. Also known as resistance training, progressive resistance training, or weight training.

tendon: A cord of connective tissue tethered at one end to muscle and at the other end to bone.

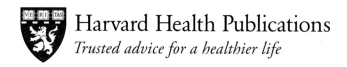

Harvard Health Publications
Trusted advice for a healthier life

 Receive *HEALTHbeat*, Harvard Health Publications' free email newsletter

Go to: **www.health.harvard.edu** to subscribe to *HEALTHbeat*. This free weekly email newsletter brings you health tips, advice, and information on a wide range of topics.

You can also join in discussion with experts from Harvard Health Publications and folks like you on a variety of health topics, medical news, and views by reading the Harvard Health Blog (**www.health.harvard.edu/blog**).

Order this report and other publications from Harvard Medical School

online | **www.health.harvard.edu**

phone | **877-649-9457** (toll-free)

mail | **Belvoir Media Group**
Attn: Harvard Health Publications
P.O. Box 5656
Norwalk, CT 06856-5656

Licensing, bulk rates, or corporate sales

email | **HHP_licensing@hms.harvard.edu**

online | **www.content.health.harvard.edu**

Other publications from Harvard Medical School

Special Health Reports *Harvard Medical School publishes in-depth reports on a wide range of health topics, including:*

Addiction	Exercise Your Joints	Positive Psychology
Allergies	Eye Disease	Prostate Disease
Advance Care Planning	Foot Care	Reducing Sugar & Salt
Aging Successfully	Grief & Loss	Rheumatoid Arthritis
Alzheimer's Disease	Hands	Sensitive Gut
Anxiety & Stress Disorders	Headache	Sexuality
Back Pain	Hearing Loss	Six-Week Eating Plan
Balance	Heart Disease	Skin Care
Caregiving	Heart Disease & Diet	Sleep
Change Made Easy	High Blood Pressure	Strength Training
Cholesterol	Incontinence	Stress Management
COPD	Knees & Hips	Stretching
Core Workout	Living Longer	Stroke
Gentle Core Workout	Memory	Thyroid Disease
Depression	Men's Health	Vitamins & Minerals
Diabetes	Neck Pain	Walking for Health
Diabetes & Diet	Nutrition	Weight Loss
Energy/Fatigue	Osteoarthritis	Women's Health
Erectile Dysfunction	Osteoporosis	Workout Workbook
Exercise	Pain Relief	Yoga

Periodicals *Monthly newsletters and annual publications, including:*

Harvard Health Letter	*Harvard Heart Letter*	*Prostate Disease Annual*
Harvard Women's Health Watch	*Harvard Men's Health Watch*	

ISBN 978-1-61401-131-6

2 8 0 0 0

9 781614 011316

ISBN 978-1-61401-131-6
SW28000

ASPT0217